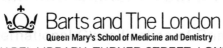

Oxford University Press makes no representation, express or implied, that the drug dosages in this book are correct. Readers must therefore always check the product information and clinical procedures with the most up to date published product information and data sheets provided by the manufacturers and the most recent codes of conduct and safety regulations. The authors and the publishers do not accept responsibility or legal liability for any errors in the text or for the misuse or misapplication of material in this work.

ICPC-2-R

International Classification of Primary Care

Revised Second Edition

Prepared by the International Classification Committee of WONCA,
the World Organization of Family Doctors.

With a CD-ROM:
ICPC in the Amsterdam Transition Project

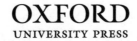

OXFORD
UNIVERSITY PRESS

OXFORD
UNIVERSITY PRESS

Great Clarendon Street, Oxford OX2 6DP

Oxford University Press is a department of the University of Oxford.
It furthers the University's objective of excellence in research, scholarship,
and education by publishing worldwide in

Oxford New York

Auckland Cape Town Dar es Salaam Hong Kong Karachi
Kuala Lumpur Madrid Melbourne Mexico City Nairobi
New Delhi Shanghai Taipei Toronto

With offices in

Argentina Austria Brazil Chile Czech Republic France Greece
Guatemala Hungary Italy Japan South Korea Poland Portugal
Singapore Switzerland Thailand Turkey Ukraine Vietnam

Oxford is a registered trade mark of Oxford University Press
in the UK and in certain other countries

Published in the United States
by Oxford University Press Inc., New York

First published 1998
Reprinted 1999, 2002
Reprinted with revisions 2005 (twice)

Okkes IM, Oskam SK, Lamberts H. ICPC in the Amsterdam Transition Project.
CD-Rom. Amsterdam: Academic Medical Center / University of Amsterdam,
Department of Family Medicine, 2005

A catalogue record for this title is available from the British Library

Library of Congress Cataloging in Publication Data
(Data available)

ISBN 0 19 8568576

978-019-856857-5

Typeset by Cepha Imaging Pvt. Ltd., Bangalore, India
Printed in Great Britain
on acid-free paper by Ashford Colour Press Ltd

Contents

The WONCA International Classification Committee (1998)

C. BRIDGES-WEBB, Chairman, Sydney, Australia
B. BENTSEN, Oslo, Norway
N. BENTZEN, Odense, Denmark
R. BERNSTEIN, Ottawa, Canada
N. BOOTH, Newcastle, UK
S. BRAGE, Oslo, Norway
H. BRITT, Sydney, Australia
L. CULPEPPER, Boston, USA
G. FISCHER, Hannover, Germany
T. GARDNER, Dunedin, New Zealand
J. GERVAS, Madrid, Spain
A. GRIMSMO, Surnadal, Norway
J. HUMBERT, Beauvoir sur Mer, France
M. JAMOULLE, Jumet, Belgium
M. KLINKMAN, Michigan, USA
M. KVIST, Turku, Finland
H. LAMBERTS, Amsterdam, The Netherlands
A. LEE, Shatin, Hong Kong
M. LIUKKO, Helsinki, Finland
I. MARSHALL, Mallorca, Spain
F. MENNERAT, Paris, France
L. MICHENER, Durham, USA
G. MILLER, Sydney, Australia
M. MIRZA, Lahore, Pakistan
S. MOHAN, Vijayawada, India
J. NUNES, Mem Martins, Portugal
I. OKKES, Amsterdam, The Netherlands
G. PARKERSON, Durham, USA
W. PATTERSON, Edinburgh, Scotland
M. RAJAKUMAR, Kuala Lumpur, Malaysia
D. SALTMAN, Sydney, Australia
P. SIVE, Herzlia, Israel
M. WOOD, Roseland, USA
T. YAMADA, Gifu, Japan
G. ZORZ, Ljubljana, Slovenia

Current Chair (2005):
Professor Niels Bentzen
Department of Community Medicine and General Practice
Norwegian University of Science and Technology
7489 Trondheim
Norway

Tel: +47 7359 8885
Fax: +47 7359 7851
E-mail: Niels.Bentzen@medisin.ntnu.no

Foreword

Increasing health care information needs are being recognized all over the world. In order to deliver optimal health care, professionals need information about the epidemiological situation in their community, diagnostic tools based on patients' reasons for encounters, and best practice information for the diagnosis and the interventions that follow. The amount of information is huge and needs to be ordered in a way that allows intuitive searches.

The International Classification of Primary Care (ICPC) is internationally the most widely used tool for ordering clinical information in primary care and family medicine. ICPC is developed and updated by the Wonca International Classification Committee (WICC) which consists of a group of practicing primary care doctors and academics. This combination of orientation on practical work and research, and the active, open minded attitude of the group is the best guarantee for the continuous development of ICPC.

The co-operation between WONCA and the World Health Organization (WHO) has a long tradition. Although the classification work originally has common roots, because of some disputes around the development of ICD and ICPC, the WHO's International Classification of Diseases in its 10th revision (ICD-10) and the second revision of ICPC (ICPC-2) have been running independently. Therefore, it was a major step forward when the WHO Family of International Classifications (WHO-FIC) network in October 2003 accepted ICPC-2 as a related classification to be used in primary care. The network also decided that a continuous co-operation between WICC and WHO-FIC network is necessary as an integral part of the revision process of ICD towards ICD-11.

WHO has expanded the scope of its classification work in the WHO-FIC system because the backbone of health care information systems is supported by three reference classifications - ICD for health problems, ICF (International Classification of Functioning, Disability and Health) for functional aspects of health, and ICHI for international classification of health care interventions.

ICPC was originally developed as a reason for encounter classification. Since a patient's reason for encounter may be a known disease, a functional health problem, or a request for an intervention, ICPC needs to cover all three reference classifications on the level of a single primary care provider. Therefore, ICPC has codes for functioning and for interventions, although it has been mainly used in the diagnostic area.

The need for coding systems has been questioned by the developers of the terminological systems. For international use one of the main problems is translation. Terms are language specific and, therefore, a detailed classification of concepts tends to be difficult to translate. For primary care, the main information needs are covered by ICPC which is already available in over 20 languages. This creates an international framework that allows international exchange of information.

Most information systems have been developed in and for developed countries. The role of developing countries in this process is important because of the information paradox in world health care: countries with the least information about the population's health face the worst health care problems. Although ICPC has been mainly developed in industrialized countries, the basic principle of a limited number of high frequency problems is applicable for any primary care setting. Modified modules may be necessary, for example for tropical conditions.

This revised edition of ICPC-2 is based on the electronic version of ICPC-2 (ICPC-2-E) which has been continuously updated since ICPC-2 was published as a book (1998). It includes all the corrections made by WICC, while most translations are already based on this version.

The availability of this updated version of the book is therefore an important milestone.

Martti Virtanen
Head of Centre, Classification expert, Pediatrician
Nordic Centre for Classifications in Healthcare
WHO-FIC network collaborating centre
Member of WICC since 1998

1 Introduction

Historical background

Until the mid-1970s most morbidity data collected in primary care research were classified using the International Classification of Diseases (ICD).[1,2] This had the important advantage of international recognition, aiding comparability of data from different countries. However, there was the disadvantage that the many symptoms and non-disease conditions that present in primary care were difficult to code with this classification, originally designed for application to mortality statistics and with a disease-based structure.

The following early references deal with some of the issues, developments and ideas about general practice classifications in the period before and after the formation of the WONCA Classification Committee in 1972:

- Research Committee of Royal College of General Practitioners. A classification of disease. *J. Roy. Coll. Gen. Pract.* 1959; **2**: 140–59.
- Westbury R C, Tarrant M. Classification of disease in general practice: a comparative study. *Can. Med. Assoc. J.* 1969; **101**: 82–7.
- Bentsen B G. Illness and general practice: a survey of medical care in an inland population in South-East Norway. Oslo: Scandinavian University Books, University Press 1970; second edition 1986.
- Hutchinson I M. The Australian morbidity survey 1969–70. *Annals of General Practice* 1971; **16**: 68–72.
- Anderson J E, Leese R E M. Patient morbidity and some patterns of family practice in South-Eastern Ontario. *Can. Med. Assoc. J.* 1975; **113**: 123–6.
- Kjaer P, Mabeck C E, Olsen O M, Pederson P. Testing WONCA's classification of diseases for use in general practice (in Danish). *Ugeskrift Laeger* 1977; **139**: 1614–16.

Recognizing the problems of the ICD, and the need for an internationally recognized classification for general practice, the WONCA Classification Committee designed the International Classification of Health Problems in Primary Care (ICHPPC), first published in 1975,[3] with a second edition in 1979[4] related to the ninth revision of ICD. Although this provided a section for the classification of some undiagnosed symptoms, it was still based on the ICD structure and was still inadequate. A third edition in 1983 had added to it criteria for the use of most of the rubrics[5] greatly adding to the reliability with which it could be used, but not overcoming its deficiencies for primary care. A new classification was needed for both the patient's reason for encounter and the provider's record of the patients' problems.

At the 1978 World Health Organization (WHO) Conference on Primary Health Care in Alma Ata,[6] adequate primary health care was recognized as the key to the goal of 'health for all by the year 2000'. Subsequently both WHO and WONCA recognized that the building of appropriate primary care systems to allow the assessment and implementation of health care priorities was only possible if the right information was available to health care planners. This led to the development of new classification systems.

Later in 1978 WHO appointed what became the WHO Working Party for Development of an International Classification of Reasons for Encounter in Primary Care.[7] This group, a majority of whose members were also members of the WONCA Classification Committee, developed a Reason for Encounter Classification (RFEC)[7–9] which later became ICPC.

Reasons for encounter (RFEs) are the agreed statement of the reason(s) why a patient enters the health care system, representing the demand for care by that person. They may be symptoms or complaints (headache or fear of cancer), known diseases (flu or diabetes), requests for preventive or diagnostic services (a blood pressure check or an ECG), a request for treatment (repeat prescription), to get test results, or administrative (a medical certificate). These reasons are usually related to one or more underlying problems which the doctor formulates at the end of the encounter as the conditions that have been treated, which may or may not be the same as the reason for the encounter.

Disease classifications are designed to allow the health care providers' interpretation of a patient's health care problem to be coded in the form of an illness, disease, or injury. In contrast, a Reason for Encounter Classification focuses on data elements from the patient's perspective.[7,10,11] In this respect, it is patient-oriented rather than disease- or provider-oriented. The reason for encounter, or demand for care, given by the patient has to be clarified by the physician or other health worker before there is an attempt to interpret and assess the patient's health problem in terms of a diagnosis, or to make any decision about the process of management and care.

The working group developing the RFE classification tested its several versions in field trials. The first field trial to test the completeness and reliability of the RFEC was a pilot study carried out in The Netherlands in 1980.[8] The results obtained from this pilot study prompted further feasibility testing in 1983. This was carried out in nine countries, namely Australia, Brazil, Barbados, Hungary, Malaysia, The Netherlands, Norway, The Philippines, and The United States.[9,12,13] The entire classification was translated from English into several languages, including French, Hungarian, Norwegian, Portuguese, and Russian. The analysis of more than 90 000 reasons for encounter recorded during over 75 000 individual encounters and the collective experience of the participants resulted in the development of a more comprehensive classification.[9,12,13]

In the course of this feasibility testing it was noted that the RFEC could easily be used to classify simultaneously the reasons for encounter and two other elements of problem-oriented care, namely the process of care and the health problems diagnosed. Thus this conceptual framework allowed the evolution of the Reason for Encounter Classification into the International Classification of Primary Care.

Problems in relation to the concurrent development of ICD-10 prevented WHO from publishing the RFEC. However, WONCA was able to develop ICPC from it and publish the first edition in 1987. While ICPC-1 was much more appropriate for primary care than previous classifications based on the ICD framework, it did not include inclusion criteria for the rubrics, or any cross-referencing. It was thus in this respect less useful than the previous publication, ICHPPC-2-defined, though it referred to it as a source of inclusion criteria which could be used.

In 1985 a project began in a number of European countries to use the new classification system to produce morbidity data from general practice for national health information systems. This involved translations of the classification and comparative studies across countries. The results were published in 1993 in a book including an update of ICPC.[14]

In 1980 WONCA became a Non-Government Organization (NGO) in official relations with WHO, and joint work together since has led to a better understanding of the requirements of primary care for its own information systems and classifications within an overall framework encompassing all health services.

The International Classification of Primary Care

The International Classification of Primary Care (ICPC[†])[15] broke new ground in the world of classification when it was published in 1987 by WONCA, the World Organization of National Colleges, Academies, and Academic Associations of General Practitioners/Family Physicians, now known more briefly as the World Organization of Family Doctors. For the first time health care providers could classify, using a single classification, three important elements of the health care encounter; reasons for encounter (RFE), diagnoses or problems, and process of care. Linkage of elements permits categorization from the beginning of the encounter with RFE to its conclusion.

The new classification departed from the traditional International Classification of Disease (ICD) chapter format where the axes of its several chapters vary, from body systems (Chapters III, IV, V, VI, VII, VIII, IX, X, XI, XIII and XIV) to aetiology (Chapters I, II, XVII, XIX, XX), and to others (Chapters XV, XVI, XVIII, XXI). This mixture of axes creates confusion, since diagnostic entities can with equal logic be classified in more than one chapter, for example influenza in either the infections chapter or the respiratory chapter, or both. Instead of conforming to this format, the ICPC chapters are all based on body systems, following the principle that localization has precedence over aetiology. The components that are part of each chapter permit considerable specificity for all three elements of the encounter, yet their symmetrical structure and frequently uniform numbering across all chapters facilitate usage even in manual recording systems. The rational and comprehensive structure of ICPC is a compelling reason to consider the classification a model for future international classifications.

Since publication, ICPC has gradually received increasing world recognition as an appropriate classification for general/family practice and primary care, and has been used extensively in some parts of the world, notably in Europe[14] and Australia.[16]

More recently the WONCA Classification Committee has participated in the international development of further initiatives related to classification, including functional

---

[†]ICPC was first published in 1987.[14] This is now referred to as ICPC-1. In 1993 it was included in a publication about its use in Europe.[13] This is referred to as ICPC-E. The 1998 publication is referred to as ICPC-2, and this revision as ICPC-2-R. ICPC is used when referring to the generic classification.

status measures, severity of illness indicators, and an international glossary for general/
family practice. Information about these is included in this book.

Classification, nomenclature, and thesaurus

Labelling aspects of general/family practice, such as reasons for encounter and health
problems, requires that the available labels reflect the characteristics of the domain:
general practice/family medicine. Labels should be derived from a nomenclature or
thesaurus. A nomenclature contains all the terms and professional jargon of medicine,
and a thesaurus is a storehouse of terms like an encyclopaedia or computer tape with a
large index and synonyms.[17]

Classification systems provide a structure to order named objects in classes according to established criteria. They do not necessarily contain all terms, and difficulties
arise when they are used as a nomenclature and terms are not found within them. Often
many terms are included within one rubric, so that the use of coding based on a classification does not provide adequate specificity.[17]

ICPC is a classification which reflects the characteristic distribution and content of
aspects of primary care. It is not a nomenclature. The richness of medicine at the level of
the individual patient needs a nomenclature and thesaurus much more extensive than
ICPC, particularly for recording the specific detail required in an individual patient record.
The use of ICPC together with ICD-10 and other classification systems, such as the
Anatomical-Therapeutic-Chemical classification of medications (ATC), can provide the
basis of an adequate nomenclature and thesaurus, but if full coding is required these must
be supplemented by even more specific coding systems. However, unless such coding
systems are based upon a suitable classification, such as ICPC is for general/family practice,
it is not possible to extract coherent data about populations rather than just individuals.[17]

Over the years there have been frictions in the relation between the available primary
care classifications (ICHPPC and ICPC) and ICD because of conceptual and taxonomi-
cal problems. ICD-10, however, now provides a widely recognized nomenclature of
diseases and health problems suitable for primary care. Although ICD-10 is not the
most appropriate tool for a primary care classification,[18] its use with ICPC as the ordering principle opens a route to good computer-based patient records allowing for the
exchange of patient data with other specialists and hospitals.[17]

ICPC-2

This second edition of ICPC has been prepared for two main reasons; to relate it to the
tenth edition of ICD, ICD-10, published by WHO in 1992,[2] and to add inclusion criteria
and cross-referencing for many of the rubrics. The latter are explained in Chapter 6 and
detailed in the tabular list in Chapter 10. In the interests of stability and consistency
very few changes to the classification have been made, though many have been suggested,
and will be the subject of ongoing work by the WONCA Classification Committee.
Feedback from users to assist this process is specially requested.

At the same time this second edition includes information about new developments in
the conceptual basis of understanding general/family practice which have arisen

in large part from the use of a classification appropriate to the discipline. These are outlined in Chapters 2–5. The book is based on the use of standard terminology as defined in the international glossary published by the WONCA Classification Committee in 1995.[19]

The book also includes information about a number of new initiatives related to classification. The Duke/WONCA Severity of Illness Checklist (DUSOI/WONCA) enables either individual health problems, or the combined health problems of the patient, to be graded in terms of severity (Chapter 7). The COOP/WONCA functional status assessment charts allow assessment of functional status of the patient independent of any particular reason for encounter or health problem (Chapter 8).

The alphabetical index to the tabular list (Chapter 12) is limited to terms from the rubric titles and their inclusion terms. It is not meant to be fully comprehensive (see Chapter 2).

ICPC and ICD

ICPC has always been linked with the widely recognized and used International Classification of Diseases published by the World Health Organization. The first edition contained a list of conversion codes to ICD-9. Since then ICD-10 has been introduced, and ICPC-2 has been carefully mapped to ICD-10 so that conversion systems can be used (Chapter 11). Users who still require a conversion to ICD-9 may obtain a disc from the WONCA Classification Committee. Extensive empirical research has confirmed that ICPC and ICD are complementary rather than in competition.

Translations

WONCA is an international organization and wishes to promote versions of ICPC in languages other than English, which is the working language of the Classification Committee. ICPC has already been translated into 19 languages, and has been published as a book in some of these (Table 1).[13,20,21] There are already several

Table 1. Availability of ICPC in different languages[17]

Basque	Hungarian
Danish+	Italian
Dutch+	Japanese+
English+	Norwegian+
Finnish+	Polish
French+	Portuguese+
German	Russian
Greek+	South African
Hebrew	Spanish+
	Swedish

+A separate edition exists in these languages.

translations of ICPC-2 being undertaken. The committee encourages anyone wishing to promote, assist with, or undertake translations of ICPC-2 to contact them to arrange cooperative work.

The WONCA policy on ICPC-2 translations is:

1. WONCA encourages versions in languages other than English.
2. These must include the whole book, not just the rubrics.
3. There must be no changes to the rubrics. Any extensions must be clearly indicated as such, and approved by the WONCA Classification Committee prior to publication.
4. Translations must be prepared by named translators working in cooperation with the WONCA Classification Committee and to the standards that it sets, particularly in relation to the extent of back translation for checking which may be required.
5. While WONCA will retain the copyright it will usually grant without fee the rights to translating organizations to retain royalties on their versions. This will require a formal agreement between WONCA and the organization or publisher concerned.

Policy on copyright and licensing

The copyright of ICPC, both in hard copy and in electronic form, is owned by WONCA. This policy relates to the electronic version and has the following aims.

Aims

1. To allow the WONCA Classification Committee to promote, distribute, and support ICPC-2, and further develop it as the best classification for primary care.
2. To maintain international comparability of versions of ICPC-2.
3. To obtain feedback and maintain a clearing-house of international experiences with ICPC-2.
4. To achieve recognition of WONCA's initiative and expertise in classification.
5. To promote understanding of appropriate links between ICPC-2 and other classification and coding systems, particularly ICD-10.
6. To encourage use of ICPC-2 rather than inhibit it with restrictions.
7. To obtain financial support to enable achievement of these aims and allow the work of the WONCA Classification Committee to continue and expand.

Policy

1. The electronic version of ICPC-2 should be made available in as many countries as possible.
2. Versions involving additions, translations, or alterations should be made with input from and agreement of the WONCA Classification Committee if they are to be regarded as official WONCA versions.
3. WONCA should license appropriate organizations to promote and distribute electronic versions of ICPC-2 in countries, regions, and language groups.
4. Licence fees may be charged through these organizations to the end users and collected by the distributors for WONCA. The fees will be set by negotiation and may be waived when there are advantages to WONCA by so doing, such as when use is for research or development.

Readers wishing to obtain this book in electronic form, or incorporate electronic versions of ICPC in computer systems, or develop and use ICPC in other ways should contact a local member of the WONCA Classification Committee (see p. vii) or WONCA (see below).

Abbreviations

As far as possible abbreviations have not been used in this book. In a few places abbreviations which are more commonly used in English than the full expansion, and which are clear in the context, are included in the rubrics. However, some have been needed, and these are as follows:

abn   abnormal
dis   disease
complt   complaint
excl   excludes
incl   includes
NOS   not otherwise specified
sympt   symptom
/   or

User feedback

In order to continue to develop ICPC the WONCA Classification Committee would like to have feedback from as many users as possible with suggestions for clarification, alterations, or extensions. Please contact a local member of the committee (see p. *vii*) or the Chair (see p. *viii*), or WONCA Executive: ceo@wonca.com.sg.

2   The structure of ICPC

ICPC is based on a simple bi-axial structure: 17 chapters based on body systems on one axis, each with an alpha code, and seven identical components with rubrics bearing a two-digit numeric code as the second axis (Fig. 1 and Table 2).

ICPC has a significant mnemonic quality which facilitates its day-to-day use by physicians, and simplifies the centralized manual coding of data recorded elsewhere.

It is presented as a tabular list (Chapter 10). The rubrics for components 1 and 7 are given in full for each chapter. The rubrics in components 2 to 6 are uniform across all chapters and are set out only once. Each rubric has a three-digit code number, a title of limited length, and the codes of the corresponding ICD-10 rubrics. Most rubrics also have inclusion terms, exclusion terms, and 'consider' terms (see Chapter 6). Abbreviations have been used sparingly, and are listed on p. 6. When the word 'multiple' is used in ICPC this refers to three or more.

The alphabetical index to the tabular list (Chapter 12) contains terms from all the rubric titles and their inclusion terms. It is not meant to be fully comprehensive; the terms included are only those which are common or important in primary care.

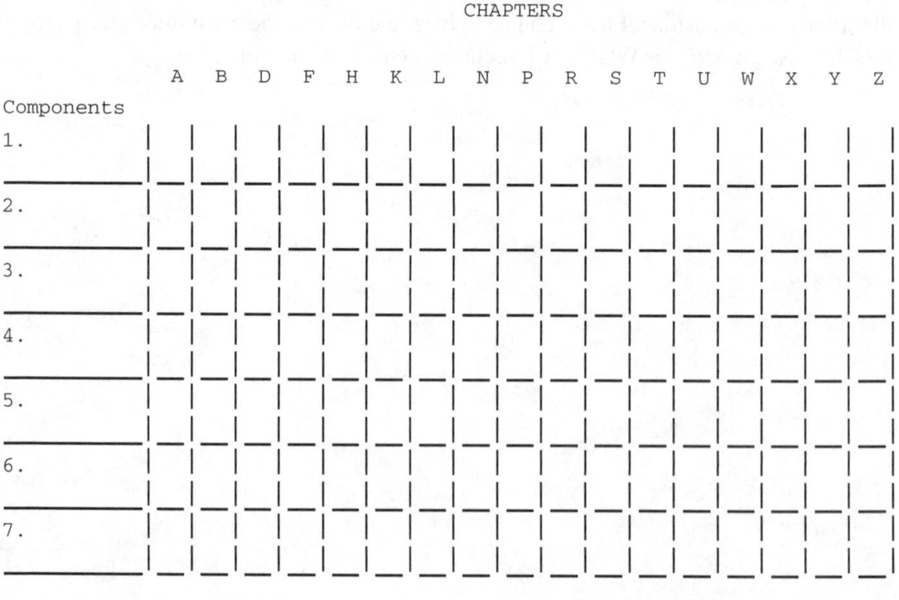

Fig. 1. The structure of ICPC: 17 chapters and 7 components.

Table 2. ICPC chapters and components

A	General and unspecified
B	Blood, blood-forming organs and immune mechanism (spleen, bone marrow)
D	Digestive
F	Eye
H	Ear (Hearing)
K	Circulatory
L	Musculoskeletal (Locomotion)
N	Neurological
P	Psychological
R	Respiratory
S	Skin
T	Endocrine, metabolic and nutritional
U	Urological
W	Pregnancy, child-bearing, family planning (Women)
X	Female genital (X.-chromosome)
Y	Male genital (Y-chromosome)
Z	Social problems

Components (standard for each chapter):

1	Complaint and symptom component
2	Diagnostic, screening, and preventive component
3	Medication, treatment, procedures component
4	Test results component
5	Administrative component
6	Referrals and other reasons for encounter
7	Disease component: —infectious diseases —neoplasms —injuries —congenital anomalies —other

A mnemonic alpha code has been used where possible.

Users seeking terms not included could use the ICD-10 index to find the ICD-10 rubric, and then the conversion tables (Chapter 11) to find the ICPC rubric. A fuller thesaurus in electronic form has been developed by some users, but an approved international version is yet to be developed.

While ICPC is comprehensive enough to allow classification of the main elements of primary care, it still has some limitations. The rubrics in components 2 to 6 covering the process of care are very broad and non-specific. A classification of medications and drugs was developed for and is described in the report of the European study,[14] but is not yet formally included. ICPC does not include objective findings found during physical examination or investigations. These are all matters for further development.

Residual rubrics

Residual rubrics ('rag-bags') are found at the end of a section or subsection; their description includes the word 'other'. Clearly, not otherwise specified (NOS) is implied for all of the terms in these rubrics. Knowledge of the boundaries of each section or subsection is required for the best use of the classification. If in doubt, consult the alphabetical index.

The practical use of morbidity/diagnostic data

Until recently classifications were mainly used for the collection of data for health statistics and formulation of policy. The advent of computer-based medical records has led to even more widespread use as a means of organizing and storing data gathered during routine clinical encounters. These data are needed both as part of the patient medical record and for extraction for health statistics. The classification and coding requirements for those two purposes differ; patient medical records require as much specific detail as possible, whereas health statistics require data which are systematically aggregated into categories based on their frequency or their importance for policy. ICPC was developed for the latter purpose, and must be modified for coding clinical data in medical records.

Optional hierarchical expansion

Clearly, no single international classification can fulfil every need for every user; inevitably users will sometimes want to separate certain problems contained in a single rubric. This usually requires expanded codes using the principle of optional hierarchy. A great deal of expansion is usually needed for coding clinical data in medical records.

It is recommended that whenever possible such expansions conform to the usage in ICD-10, or that ICD-10 codes are used as expansion codes, so that maximum comparability between data systems is maintained. Even then provision for including patient-specific text is needed for adequate specificity for patient care records.[17]

Severity of illness and functional status

Information about severity of illness and functional status assessment of the patient may be recorded in association with use of ICPC, and means of classifying these are therefore included in this book. The Duke/WONCA Severity of Illness Checklist (DUSOI/WONCA) can be related to ICPC rubrics and may be applied to individual health problems, as well as being summed to indicate the severity of the patient's combined health problems (Chapter 7). The COOP/WONCA functional status assessment charts apply to the patient independent of his/her health problems, and are explained in Chapter 8.

3   Episode of care: a central concept of general/family practice

Changes in the need for and use of classifications in primary care have continued since the publication of ICPC in 1987. The main purpose of the classification was then seen to be its use in gathering data for research and policy formulation. However, its use has now widened as research data and practical experiences with ICPC, as well as the emergence of new concepts in general/family medicine, have resulted in new applications.

The most important new applications of the use of ICPC are in describing the construct of episodes of care and in computer patient records. The two are closely related, and depend upon the use of ICPC as the ordering principle of patient data gathered in general/family practice and primary care.

The WONCA definition of general/family practice refers to 'a physician who provides personal, primary, and continuing comprehensive health care to individuals and families'.[19] This is quite similar to that of primary care in the new Institute of Medicine (IOM) definition: 'Primary care is the provision of integrated accessible health care services by clinicians who are accountable for addressing a large majority of personal health care needs, developing a sustained partnership with patients and practising in the context of family and community'.[22]

Episode of care

These definitions have been made operational by choosing the 'episode of care' as the appropriate unit of assessment. Episodes of care are distinguished from episodes of illness or disease in a population. An episode of care is a health problem or disease from its first presentation to a health care provider until the completion of the last encounter for that same health problem or disease (Fig. 2).[17]

Reasons for encounter, health problems/diagnoses, and process of care/interventions form the core of an episode of care consisting of one or more encounters, including changes in their relations over time ('transitions'). An episode of care, consequently, refers to all care provided for a discrete health problem or disease in a particular patient. The 'large majority of personal health care needs', the 'comprehensiveness', the degree of 'integration', of 'accessibility', and of 'accountability' can be assessed when episodes of care are classified with ICPC in a computer-based patient record.

Start of episode

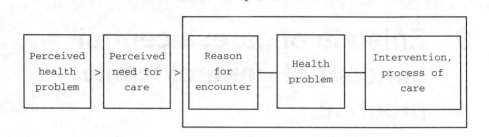

Second encounter of same episode

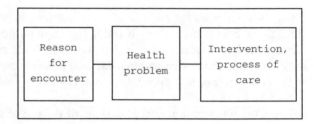

Fig. 2. An episode of care.

The use of the concept of episode of care was demonstrated in the European study using ICPC.[14] In this study, characteristic epidemiological and clinical similarities and differences between the various sites were established. Also, the concept of reason for encounter proved to be an innovative and practical operationalization of the patient's perspective and demand for care; the validity of the reason for encounter as it was coded by family doctors when compared with the patient's point of view after the encounter, was consistently very high.[23]

The new International Glossary of Primary Care defines the content of general/family practice and gives rules to structure episodes with ICPC in order to allow epidemiological standard retrievals, and to make them comparable in different countries.[19]

Reason for encounter

The reason for encounter (RFE) has been established to be a practical source of patient information, also useful for research and education. This is illustrated by epidemiological data from the Dutch Transition project in the form of standard output, following the rules of the glossary.[17] Beginning with the reason for encounter allows the determination of the probabilities of any given health problem at the start or during follow-up of the episode, per standard sex age group. Thus the top 10 problems related to cough at the start of an episode show clinically important differences between children aged 5–14 and

Table 3. Top 10 episode titles starting with cough (R05) as the reason for encounter (prior probabilities)

RFE R05 Cough (*N* = 1267)	*N*	*%*
R74 URI (head cold)	456	35.6
R78 Acute bronchitis/bronchiolitis	261	20.4
R05 Cough	159	12.4
R77 Acute laryngitis/tracheitis	110	8.6
A77 Other viral diseases NOS	54	4.2
R96 Asthma	40	3.1
R81 Pneumonia	33	2.6
R75 Sinusitis acute/chronic	30	2.3
R80 Influenza without pneumonia	24	1.9
R71 Whooping cough	22	1.7
Total top 10	1189	92.8
Total	1281	100.0
Men aged 65–74 (*N* = 646)	*N*	*%*
R78 Acute bronchitis/bronchiolitis	256	39.1
R74 URI (head cold)	155	23.7
R05 Cough	65	9.9
R77 Acute laryngitis/tracheitis	45	6.9
R75 Sinusitis acute/chronic	22	3.4
K77 Heart failure	15	2.3
R96 Asthma	13	2.0
R91 Chronic bronchitis/bronchiectasis	12	1.8
R81 Pneumonia	10	1.5
R95 Emphysema/COPD	9	1.4
Total top 10	602	92.0
Total	654	100.0

Source: Transition Project, reported in Hofmans-Okkes and Lamberts.[17]

men aged 65–74 (Table 3). The reverse procedure is equally relevant from a clinical point of view: what reasons for encounter were presented at the start and during follow-up of a problem in each standard sex age group? This is illustrated for acute bronchitis (Table 4). These tables document the clinical differences in far more detail than has been possible until now.

The health problem/diagnosis

The health problem/diagnosis is central to the episode of care and gives it its name. Many health problems are in fact medical diagnoses, but many in primary care are other conditions such as fear of disease, symptoms, complaints, disabilities, or need for care

Table 4. Top 10 reasons for encounter in an episode of acute bronchitis/bronchiolitis (R78)

Children aged 5–14 ($N = 377$)	N	%
R05 Cough	321	46.1
A03 Fever	98	14.1
R31 Med exam/health evalua/partial	64	9.2
R02 Shortness of breath/dyspnoea	43	6.2
R74 URI (head cold)	24	3.4
A04 General weakness/tiredness	18	2.6
R03 Wheezing	17	2.4
R64 Provide init episode new/ongoing	17	2.4
R78 Acute bronchitis/bronchiolitis	13	1.9
R21 Sympt/complt throat	9	1.3
Total top 10	624	89.5
Total	697	100.0
Men aged 65–74 ($N = 422$)	**N**	**%**
R05 Cough	324	39.4
R02 Shortness of breath/dyspnoea	133	16.2
R78 Acute bronchitis/bronchiolitis	100	12.2
R31 Med exam/health evalua/partial	79	9.6
A03 Fever	34	4.1
R25 Abnormal sputum/phlegm	23	2.8
R64 Provide init episode new/ongoing	21	2.6
R74 URI (head cold)	14	1.7
A04 General weakness/tiredness	13	1.6
R01 Pain attrib to respir system	8	1.0
Total top 10	749	91.1
Total	822	100.0

Source: Transition Project, reported in Hofmans-Okkes and Lamberts.[17]

such as immunization. ICPC includes all of these. The health problem may be qualified in terms of its status in the encounter, the certainty which the provider assigns to its diagnosis, and its severity.

The status of the episode in an encounter can be specified as new to both doctor and patient, new to doctor but previously treated outside the current provider system, or neither in the case of follow-up encounters (Fig. 3D). A good computer patient record warns the provider when s/he tries to enter a follow-up encounter for an episode that has not yet been established in the database, or whenever a new one is started when an episode with the same title already exists. This is, obviously, vital to ensure the quality of day to day recording.

The extent to which the doctor is certain that his or her diagnosis is correct is another aspect of an episode of care; this can be graded from uncertain to certain, but a standard

The old structure

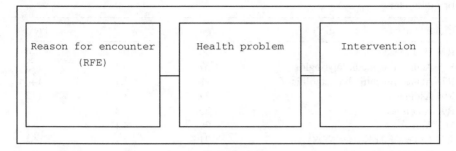

The new structure

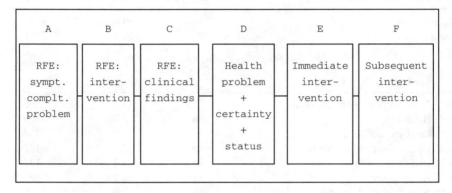

Fig. 3. A new structure for describing encounters.[17]

means of doing this has not yet been adopted. The inclusion criteria for use of rubrics in ICPC-2 will, however, help to ensure that the label chosen for the episode is used consistently by all providers. Pop-up screens can be used to display options at the time of coding in computer-based records.

The third qualification of an episode of care, severity, is discussed in Chapter 7.

Patients with multiple health problems and episodes of care are common in primary care. A good data system will be able to display the interrelationships of these, and provide data on comorbidity (Table 5).

Interventions, the process of care

The specificity of the three-digit ICPC process code to classify immediate interventions is limited, but usually adequate. However, when drugs are prescribed a drug code is needed. Because of the vast number of medications involved, and the idiosyncrasies of national drug availabilities, no internationally suitable code has yet been produced.

Table 5. Comorbid episodes for patients with R78, acute bronchitis/bronchiolitis

Children aged 5–14 ($N = 329$)	N	%	Prev.
R74 URI (head cold)	90	9.6	274
R71 Acute otitis media/myringitis	57	6.1	173
R78 Acute bronchitis/bronchiolitis	48	5.1	146
R96 Asthma	37	3.9	112
R97 No disease	32	3.4	97
S03 Warts	29	3.1	88
A77 Other viral diseases NOS	21	2.2	64
R76 Tonsillitis acute	20	2.1	61
S18 Laceration/cut	20	2.1	61
D73 Presumed GI infection	17	1.8	52
Total top 10	371	39.6	1128
Total	938	100.0	2851

Mean number of comorbid episodes = 2.9

Men aged 65–74 ($N = 350$)	N	%	Prev.
R78 Acute bronchitis/bronchiolitis	72	4.7	206
A97 No disease	56	3.7	160
R95 Emphysema/COPD	47	3.1	134
K86 Uncomplicated hypertension	46	3.0	131
R74 URI (head cold)	46	3.0	131
K77 Heart failure	35	2.3	100
A85 Adv effect med agent proper dose	30	2.0	86
H81 Excessive ear wax	30	2.0	86
K76 Other/chron ischemic heart dis	30	2.0	86
T90 Diabetes mellitus	25	1.6	71
Total top 10	417	27.4	1191
Total	1521	100.0	4346

Mean number of comorbid episodes = 4.3

Prev. = Number of comorbid episodes per 1000 patients with R78.
Source: Transition Project, reported in Hofmans-Okkes and Lamberts.[17]

In Europe an ICPC drug code which is ATC compatible has been valuable and may be suitable for wider adoption.[13]

Patient records

The core of a computer-based patient record is data coded with ICPC which is language independent: this enhances the use of practice records for a comparison of data from different countries, and it supports the development of general/family practice as an internationally well developed profession with a well defined and empirically based frame of reference. The availability of ICPC in 19 languages and the growing number of translations of ICD-10 accompanied by alphabetical indexes will allow family doctors in many countries to incorporate a detailed language-specific thesaurus in their system, at the same time using ICPC to systematically structure their records and the database in a more standardized way.

Further developments

The original three basic elements of encounters to be coded with ICPC (reason for encounter, health problem, and interventions) (Fig. 2) have now been expanded into six data entry options (A–F) for computer-based patient records (Fig. 3).[17] The reason for encounter is recorded in two sections: the patient's symptoms and complaints, and the patient's requests for interventions. The clinical findings elicited by the physician in the form of symptoms and complaints are coded in addition to those presented as reasons for encounter. Interventions or processes of care are recorded as immediate (those occurring during the encounter) or subsequent (those which will be done subsequently). Work with these, particularly in The Netherlands, has confirmed the usefulness of the concept of reason for encounter, and further refined the concepts of reason for encounter, health problem/diagnosis, and process of care.[14]

The use of reasons for encounter to estimate prior probabilities is clearly very useful; it can be even more so if reasons for encounter presented by the patient such as cough, shortness of breath, fever, abnormal sputum, or wheezing (Fig. 3A) are distinguished from clinical findings elicited by the physician during history taking (Fig. 3C). ICPC incorporates over 200 symptoms and complaints serving the classification of reasons for encounter and of clinical findings equally well, though it should be noted that it does not yet include a classification of objective findings. Both applications can be included in the encounter and episode structure of a computer-based patient record (Fig. 3A and C). Together they allow a complete calculation of prior probabilities, while the difference between a symptom expressed by the patient as a reason for encounter or elicited by the physician is retained, and the probabilities can be calculated separately if required.

Reasons for encounter in the form of symptoms, complaints or health problems/ diagnoses should be distinguished explicitly from those in the form of requests for interventions such as a prescription, an X-ray, a referral, or advice (Fig. 3A and B). Requests for a certain intervention are often followed by this intervention being performed: when patients ask for medication or a blood test, they often receive it.[17] Since patients do actively influence the care provided by general practitioners/family doctors it is important to explicitly document this, also to obtain a better understanding of compliance.

Recording systems should be able to distinguish between diagnostic and therapeutic interventions during the encounter ('immediate', Fig. 3E) and those that will follow ('subsequent', Fig. 3F). The difference between what is in fact being done by the family doctor at the time of the encounter and what is expected to follow is important for the analysis of utilization data, interdoctor variation, and compliance. It also allows better understanding of the shift from prior probabilities in the first encounter of an episode of care to the posterior probabilities during follow-up.[17]

For recording subsequent interventions a more specific process classification than ICPC provides is needed. Development of this is an ongoing activity of the WONCA Classification Committee.

4 Use of ICPC for recording reason for encounter

Procedures for coding information using ICPC vary somewhat according to the type of information being recorded, for example reason for encounter, health problem, or intervention. In order to promote consistent recording and therefore better comparability of data between centres, the following standards are suggested.

Reason for encounter

The primary care provider should identify and clarify the reason for the encounter (RFE) as stated by the patient without making any judgments as to the correctness or accuracy of the reason. This use of the classification is guided by three principles:

1. The reason for encounter should be understood and agreed upon between the patient and the provider and should be recognized by the patient as an acceptable description.
2. The ICPC rubric chosen should be as close as possible to the original statement of the reason given by the patient and must represent a minimal or no transformation by the provider. However, clarification of the patient's reasons for encounter within the framework of ICPC is necessary so that the most appropriate rubric in the classification can be applied.
3. The inclusion criteria listed for rubrics for use in recording health problems/diagnoses are NOT to be used, since the reason for encounter is to be documented from the patient's point of view, based entirely on the patient's statement of the reason.

The way in which a patient expresses his/her reason(s) for encounter determines which chapter and which component to use (Fig. 1 and Table 2). The entire classification is applicable as patients can describe their reasons for seeking health care in the form of symptoms or complaints, as requests for services, or as health problems.

Choosing the chapter code

To code the RFE it is necessary to first select the appropriate organ system or chapter, assign the correct alpha code, and then the two-digit numeric code in the relevant component such as a symptom or complaint, a diagnosis, or an intervention. The alphabetical index should be used when there is uncertainty about the chapter or component in which a specific reason for encounter should be placed. Chapter A is used for reasons for encounter which relate to unspecified or multiple body systems.

When ICPC is used for recording RFE four rules apply to the use of the chapters, and three rules to the use of components. Those rules are listed below with examples of the application of those rules.

Rule 1

The reason for the encounter should be coded as specifically as possible and may require some clarification by the provider.

Example

Chest pain can be coded as A11 (chest pain not otherwise specified (NOS)), or as KOI (pain attributed to heart), or as R01 (pain respiratory), or as L04 (chest symptoms/complaints). The decision as to the correct selection is not based on the opinion of the provider as to the type of chest pain but, rather, to the manner in which the patient expresses his/her reason for encounter when clarification is sought by the provider.

'Its all over my chest ...'	A11
'My chest hurts when I cough'	R01
'I have chest pain ... I think its my heart'	KO1
'I have chest pain after falling down stairs'	L04

Rule 2

Whenever the patient makes a specific statement use his/her terminology.

Example

Jaundice, in the form of a diagnostic descriptive term can be found in Chapter D (digestive) but the patient may present this symptom as a yellow discoloration of the skin (Chapter S). If the patient expresses the problem as 'jaundice', the ICPC code is D13. If, however, the patient states 'my skin has gone yellow' the correct code would be SOS, regardless of the fact that the health care provider is positive that the diagnosis is some form of hepatitis.

Rule 3

When the patient is unable to describe his/her complaint, the reason given by the accompanying person is acceptable as that stated by the patient (e.g. a mother bringing in a child or relatives accompanying an unconscious patient).

Rule 4

Any problem whatsoever presented verbally by the patient should be recorded as a reason for encounter. Multiple coding is required if the patient gives more than one reason. Code every reason presented at whatever stage in the encounter it occurs.

Example

'I need my blood pressure tablets. Also my breasts are tender and sore' —K50, XI8. If later the patients asks 'What is this lump on my skin?' that is also coded as a reason for encounter —S04.

Choosing the component code

1. Symptoms and complaints

The most common reasons patients give for seeking health care are presented in the form of symptoms and complaints.[14,16,23,24] Therefore, it is expected that Component 1 (symptoms and complaints) will be used extensively. These symptoms are specific for each chapter; nausea is found in the Digestive chapter (D09), while sneezing (R07) is located in the Respiratory chapter. While most of the entries in this component are symptoms specific to the chapter in which they are found, some standardization has been introduced for ease of coding.

Throughout most of the chapters, with the exception of psychological and social, the first rubric(s) relate to the symptom pain. Examples of these are earache (HOI) and headache (N01). There are also four standard Component 1 rubrics in each chapter. They are:

- 26 Fear of cancer
- 27 Fear of having a disease or condition
- 28 Limited function/disability
- 29 Other symptoms/complaints

Codes 26 and 27, and sometimes also a few others, are used when the patient expresses concern about or fear of cancer or some other condition or disease. Examples are:

'I'm afraid I have TB'	A27
'I'm worried that I have cancer of the breast'	X26
'I'm scared of venereal disease'	Y25

Even though the provider thinks that such an expressed fear is unwarranted or illogical, it constitutes the patient's reason for encounter.

Rubric —28 should be used when the patient's reason for encounter is expressed in terms of a disability which affects activities of daily life and social functions.

Examples

'I cannot climb stairs because of the cast they have put on my leg for my fractured ankle' —L28 (Component 1) and L76 (Component 7).

'I can't work in the office because I can't sit for any length of time because of my hemorrhoids' —K28 (Component 1) and K96 (Component 7).

In each chapter the component code 29 is the residual or 'rag-bag' rubric for symptoms/complaints. This contains uncommon and unusual symptoms and complaints which do not have a separate rubric, and is also appropriate for symptoms/complaints which are not clearly stated. The index should be checked for synonymous terms in other rubrics before using this rubric.

2. Diagnostic, screening and preventive procedures

The reasons included in this concept are those in which the patient seeks some sort of procedure, such as 'I'm here to have a blood test' (—34). The patient may request a particular procedure in connection with an expressed problem or as a single demand, such as

'I want the doctor to examine my heart' K31, or
'I think I need to have my urine tested' (—35), or
'I've come for the result of my X-ray'(—60), or
'I need a vaccination'(—44).

Clarification by the provider is necessary to find out why the patient thinks he or she needs a urine test in order to select the appropriate alpha code. If it is because of a possible bladder infection the code is U35; if because of diabetes T35. If the result of an X-ray which is being requested refers to a barium meal D60. A request for vaccination against rubella A44.

3. Medication, treatment, procedures

These reasons are expressed when the patient requests a treatment or when the patient refers to the physician's instructions to return for specific treatment, procedure, or medication as the reason for encounter. Further clarification by the provider is often necessary in order to identify the most appropriate code.

Examples

'I need my medication' (—50). If the patient expresses the reason why he is taking the medication or the provider knows the reason, select the appropriate alpha code, e.g. for a sinus infection the code would be R50.

'I'm here to have my cast removed' (—54). If it is evident that, for instance, the patient had a fracture of the left arm the correct alpha code to select would be L.

'I was told to come for removal of the stitches today' (—54). Although at first one might assume that all suture removal would be in the Skin chapter, the patient might have stitches from eyelid surgery F54 or from a phimosis operation Y54.

4. Test results

This component should be used when the patient is specifically requesting the results of tests previously carried out. The fact that the results of the test may be negative does not affect the use of this component. Often the patient will request the test result and its consequences and seek more information on the underlying problem. In that case, also consider using the additional code —45 (health education, advice).

Examples

'I need the results of my blood test'. If the test was for anaemia code B60, if for lipids T60, if the patient cannot specify A60.

'I want to know what they found on the X-rays of my stomach that were taken last week' (D60).

'I am supposed to pick up the result of my urine test and take it to the urologist. I also want to know what he will do and which examinations and treatment I can expect' (U60, U45).

5. Administrative

Administrative reasons for encounter with the health care system include such things as examinations required by a third party (someone other than the patient), insurance forms which require completion, and discussions regarding the transfer of records.

Examples

'I need this medical insurance form completed' (A62).

'My fracture is healed and I need a certificate to go back to work' (L62).

6. Referrals and other reasons for encounter

If the patient's reason for encounter is to be referred to another provider —66, —67, and —68 can be used for this purpose. If the patient states his/her reason for the encounter is 'being sent by someone else', use —65.

When a provider initiates a new episode or takes the initiative for the follow-up of an already existing episode of a health problem such as hypertension, obesity, alcoholism, or a smoking habit, it will be appropriate to code the reason for encounter as —64.

Example

A patient presenting with a blocked ear due to earwax, which is removed, has his blood pressure measured and found to be high, and also receives advice about smoking. The patient's reasons for encounter and the related problems and treatment would be recorded as follows:

H13 (blocked feeling in ear), H81 (earwax), H51 (removal of earwax).

K64 (provider initiated), K85 (raised blood pressure), K31 (checking of blood pressure).

P64 (provider initiated), PI7 (tobacco abuse), P45 (advice to stop smoking).

7. Diagnosis/disease

Only when the patient expresses the reason for encounter as a specific diagnosis or disease should it be coded in Component 7. The reason for encounter of a patient who is known to be a diabetic but comes in complaining of weakness should not be coded to diabetes but to the problem expressed: weakness (A04). However, if the patient states that he has come about his diabetes the diagnosis 'diabetes' should be coded as his reason for encounter (T90).

If the patient names a reason for encounter in the form of a diagnosis which the provider knows is not correct, the 'wrong' RFE of the patient is coded rather than the 'correct' one of the physician; for example a patient presenting with a reason for encounter of 'migraine', when the provider knows it is tension headache, or a patient who is known to have nasal polyps presenting with 'hayfever'.

Examples

'I am here because of my hypertension' (K86).

'I come every month for the arthritis of my hip' (L89).

Rules for components

The following rules for the use of each component will reinforce the description of the components.

Rule 1

Whenever a code is shown preceded by a dash (—), select the chapter code (alpha). Use A when no specific chapter can be selected, or when multiple chapters are involved. All codes must begin with an alpha code to be complete.

Example

Biopsy will be coded —52, for digestive system D52, for skin S52. Medication prescribed will be coded as —50. A patient requesting medication for asthma R50.

Rule 2

Rubrics from more than one component, or more than one rubric from the same component, can be used for the same encounter if more than one reason is presented by the patient.

Example

'I've had abdominal pain since last night and I vomited several times' D01, D10.

'I have some abdominal pain and I think that I may have appendicitis' D06, D88.

5 Use of ICPC for recording health problems and process of care (interventions)

Health problems

ICPC can be used to record the provider's assessment of the patient's health problems. This can be done in terms of symptoms and complaints, or diagnoses, so can be derived from Component 1 or Component 7. The latter is based on the lists of diseases, injuries, and related health problems in the International Classification of Diseases (ICD), but includes as separate rubrics only those that are common or important in primary care.

Many of the health problems which are managed in primary care cannot be designated in terms of disease or injury. They include symptoms and complaints, which are listed in Component 1. Sometimes there is no apparent health problem involved in an episode of care, as when it relates to need for immunization or a Pap smear or advice. These episodes can be labelled using rubrics such as A97 No Disease, or A98 Health Maintenance/Preventive Medicine.

In Components 1 and 7 the corresponding ICD-10 codes are listed for each rubric. Sometimes these are an exact one-to-one match, but more often there are several ICD codes for an ICPC-2 rubric, and sometimes there are several ICPC-2 codes for a single ICD-10 rubric. A full conversion structure is given in Chapter 10.

In order to improve reliability of coding health problems using ICPC-2, many of the rubrics in Component 7 have inclusion criteria specified. These are explained in Chapter 6.

Rubrics in Components 1 and 7 often have additional information as a guide to their use: lists of synonyms and alternative descriptions as inclusion terms; lists of similar conditions which should be coded elsewhere as exclusion terms; and lists of less specific codes which might be considered if the particular patient's condition does not meet the inclusion criteria. There are no such guidelines for rubrics in the process Components 2 to 6.

General rules for coding health problems

Users are encouraged to record during each encounter, the full spectrum of problems managed, including organic, psychological, and social health problems, in the form of episode(s) of care. Recording should be at the highest level of diagnostic refinement for which the user can be confident, and which meets the inclusion criteria for that rubric.

In any data system it is necessary to have clear and specific criteria for the way in which health problems or episodes of care are recorded. This applies particularly to the relationship between the underlying condition and manifestations when both may be available as rubrics in the classification, and is best illustrated by an example. A patient with ischaemic heart disease may also have atrial fibrillation and resulting anxiety. It should be policy to include as separate episodes of care manifestations which require different management, and in the above example the atrial fibrillation and anxiety would be recorded as additional episodes of care.

Some systems require that problems be coded only from components 1 and 7; others also accept codes from other components, so that if, for example, the patient attends for a tetanus immunization without a current injury, the problem could be coded as N44.

In ICPC localization within a body system takes precedence over aetiology, so that when coding a condition which because of its aetiology can be found in several chapters (for example, trauma) the appropriate chapter should be used. Chapter A (general) should be considered only if the site is not specified or if the disease affects more than two body systems. All chapters provide specific rubrics based on the body system or organ involved in the disease and the aetiology. Conditions accompanying and affecting pregnancy or the puerperium are usually coded to Chapter W, but a condition is not coded to Chapter W merely because the patient is pregnant; it should be coded to the appropriate rubric in the chapter representing the body system involved. All social problems, whether identified as a reason for encounter or as a problem, are listed in the first component of Chapter Z.

Specific rules for coding health problems using inclusion criteria (see also Chapter 6)

1. Coding of diagnoses should occur at the highest level of specificity possible for that patient encounter.
2. Inclusion criteria contain the minimum number of criteria necessary to permit coding with that rubric.
3. Consult the criteria *after* the diagnosis has been formulated. They are NOT guidelines for diagnosis, NOR are they intended to be used as a guide to therapeutic decisions.
4. If the criteria cannot be fulfilled, consult other less specific rubrics suggested by the term 'consider'.
5. For those rubrics without inclusion criteria, consult the list of inclusion terms in the rubric, and take into account any exclusion terms.

Process of care, interventions

ICPC can be used to classify the interventions used in the process of medical care with Components 2, 3, 5, and part of Component 6; however, Component 4 and some rubrics of Component 6, namely, —63, —64, —65, and —69, cannot be used in this way.

These process rubrics are broad and general, rather than specific. For instance, a blood test (—34), even if relating to only one body system (e.g. cardiovascular, K34), may encompass a great variety of different tests such as enzymes, lipids, or electrolytes.

The process codes in Components 2, 3, and 5 follow the major headings to be found in the far more detailed IC-Process-PC, which was developed by the WONCA Classification Committee.[25] ICPC and IC-Process-PC are, therefore, compatible one with the other. The details found in IC-Process-PC may be applied to the three-digit ICPC codes by expanding to four or five digits.

In Components 2, 3,5, and the part of Component 6 which can be used to classify the process of care, the rubric codes are standard throughout the chapters at the two-digit level. The alpha code of the correct chapter has to be added by the provider who is doing the coding. A limited number of rubrics in the first and seventh components of Chapters W, X, and Y also contain procedures such as delivery, abortion, and family planning.

The most important principle in the coding process is to code all those interventions which take place during that particular encounter and which have a logical relation to the episode of care. A fourth or fifth digit may be necessary for increased specificity, as in the following examples:

Example 1

—54 Repair/fixation/suture/cast/prosthetic device
L54.1 Application of casts
L54.2 Removal of casts

Example 2

—40 Diagnostic endoscopy
—D40 Diagnostic endoscopy of the digestive system
—D40.1 Gastroscopy

More than one process code may be used for each encounter, but it is extremely important to be consistent. For instance, measuring the blood pressure, which is routine for hypertension, can be coded as K31 on every occasion. Routine examinations, complete or partial, both for body systems or for the general chapter must also be coded with consistency. Below are examples of definitions for complete and partial examinations which have been used in one setting. However, it is essential that each country develops a definition of what constitutes a 'complete examination—general' and a 'complete examination—body system' for that culture and that these definitions are used consistently. This will ensure that what is contained in each 'partial examination—general' or 'partial examination—body system', in that country will also have consistency.

Complete examination

The term 'complete examination' refers to an examination which contains those elements of professional assessment which by consensus of a group of local professionals reflects the usual standard of care. This examination will be complete with regard to either the body system (e.g. eye, Chapter F) or as a complete general examination (Chapter A).

Partial examination

The term 'partial examination' in any chapter refers to a partial examination directed to the appropriate specific organ system or function. When more than two systems are involved in a limited or incomplete examination it is designated general (Chapter A). Most encounters will include a partial examination to evaluate acute and simple illnesses or return visits for chronic illnesses. The following are examples:

Complete examination—general, general check-up = A30

Complete neurological examination = N30

Partial examination—general, limited check on several body systems such as respiratory and cardiovascular = A31

Partial examination—body system, measuring blood pressure = K31

The following procedures are regarded by the WONCA Classification Committee as included in routine examinations to be coded in rubrics —30 and —31 rather than coded separately:

- inspection, palpation, percussion, auscultation
- visual acuity and fundoscopy
- otoscopy
- vibration sense (tuning fork examination)
- vestibular function (excluding calormetric tests)
- digital rectal and vaginal examination
- vaginal speculum examination
- blood pressure recording
- indirect laryngoscopy
- height/weight.

All other examinations are to be included in other rubrics.

Component 2—diagnostic, screening and preventive procedures

Diagnostic and preventive procedures cover a wide range of health care activities including immunizations, screening, risk appraisal, education, and counselling.

Component 3—medications, treatment, procedures

This component is designed to classify those procedures done on site by the primary care provider. It is not intended that it be used to document procedures done by providers to whom the patient has been referred, for which a much more extensive list of procedures would be required. Immunizations are coded in Component 2.

Component 4—test results

Component 4 does not relate to process or interventions.

Component 5—administrative

This component is designed to classify those instances where the provision of a written document or form by the provider for the patient or other agency is warranted by existing regulations, laws, or customs. Writing a referral letter is only considered to be an administrative service when it is the sole activity performed during the encounter, otherwise it is included in Component 6.

Component 6—referrals, and other reasons for encounter

Referrals to other primary care providers, physicians, hospitals, clinics, or agencies for therapeutic or counselling purposes, are to be coded in this component. Referrals for an X-ray or a laboratory investigation should be coded in Component 2.

For more specificity, a fourth digit can be added, for example:

—66 Referral to other provider/nurse/therapist/social worker.
  —66.1 Nurse
  —66.2 Physiotherapist
  —66.3 Social worker

—67 Specialist
  —67.1 Internist
  —67.2 Cardiologist
  —67.3 Surgeon.

6 Inclusion criteria in ICPC

Introduction

It has always been clear to the WONCA Classification Committee that an internationally agreed list of rubrics to classify problems met in primary care would not in itself ensure the highest level of statistical comparability. In the International Classification of Health Problems in Primary Care (ICHPPC-2-Defined) published in 1983 inclusion criteria for the use of each rubric were introduced to improve consistency of coding.[5]

Inclusion criteria are not the same as definitions. They should be considered in relation to their purpose, to improve consistency of coding, rather than as definitions for delineating health problems. We have, however, tried to ensure that they are compatible with accepted definitions, such as those in the International Nomenclature of Diseases (IND).

In this publication many of the inclusion criteria originating in ICHPPC-2-Defined have been updated and are directly related to ICPC rubrics. In some instances, new or extensively modified inclusion criteria have been created based on the theoretical framework described in the next section. Although this publication marks an advance in the taxonomy of general/family practice, it is not yet ideal. ICPC is a classification very much in evolution, and experience with the inclusion criteria presented in this volume will undoubtedly lead to further refinement in the years to come. We welcome comments from users.

Theoretical framework for assignment of inclusion criteria

The theoretical framework used to assign inclusion criteria in this classification is based on the presence of four general categories of diagnosis in primary care: aetio-logical and pathological disease entities, pathophysiological conditions, nosological diagnoses (syndromes), and symptom diagnoses. It was decided to apply different principles to each category based on its characteristics:

- *Aetiological and pathological*: the diagnosis has proven pathology or aetiology; inclusion criteria are based on standard disease definition, with modification where necessary to allow application to general/family practice. Examples: appendicitis, acute myocardial infarction.
- *Pathophysiological*: the diagnosis has a proven pathophysiological substrate; inclusion criteria include symptoms, complaints, and characteristic objective findings. Examples: presbyacusis, hypertension.
- *Nosological*: the diagnosis depends on a symptom complex based on consensus between physicians, without a proven pathological or pathophysiological base or

aetiology, and is often called a syndrome; inclusion criteria include only symptoms and complaints. Examples: depression, irritable bowel syndrome.

- *Symptom*: a symptom or complaint is the best medical label for the episode. Examples: fatigue, eye pain.

The criteria

The underlying principle used was to provide THE MOST CONCISE INCLUSION CRITERIA POSSIBLE WHICH WOULD MINIMIZE VARIABILITY IN CODING. Adherence to this principle led to the use of *minimal inclusion criteria* for each rubric. This requires further explanation.

For most diagnostic rubrics, the reader will find one or more criteria which must be fulfilled to code a problem under that title. Sometimes there is a choice of criteria; at other times criteria from a list must be met. When 'or' is used in a list it is with its inclusive meaning, which is the same as 'and/or'. 'Multiple' in this book means three or more.

Attempts were made to specify the *minimum criteria* needed in order to reduce the complexity of coding and thus minimize miscoding. In addition, we have only included those criteria which have sufficient *discriminatory value* to distinguish one rubric from another with which it might be confused. In some cases, the available criteria may be too few to exclude *all* other possible conditions which might be coded mistakenly to a particular rubric, but they will exclude the common ones.

The criteria have whenever possible been based on clinical criteria, rather than requiring the results of tests and investigations. They are as far as possible independent of technology, which varies considerably throughout the world, and is rapidly changing. This makes them appropriate for primary care use throughout the world.

This approach is very different from that seen in classic disease-oriented textbooks, which usually list all signs and symptoms, or all potential criteria, associated with a particular diagnostic title. We believe that in order to maximize the utility of criteria-based problem coding in general practice, brevity must supersede exhaustiveness.

Sometimes the rubric title is itself adequately specific. In these cases, no inclusion criteria are given. To avoid errors, each rubric, with inclusion and exclusion terms, and inclusion criteria, should be read in its entirety.

Attempts were not made to provide criteria for every rubric, particularly residual rubrics, which contain too many disparate diagnoses for useful definition. In these cases, the reader should consult the list of diagnoses included in the rubric title and inclusion terms, or refer to the more complete list given for the relevant rubrics in ICD-10.

Cross-referencing

As well as inclusion criteria, each rubric may have the following information:

- includes: a list of synonyms and alternative descriptions which are included in the rubric

- excludes: a list of similar conditions which should be coded elsewhere, with the appropriate code for each
- consider: a list of rubrics with their codes, usually less specific, which might be considered if the particular patient's condition does not meet the inclusion criteria

Advantages of this framework

The use of this framework results in clear and generally accepted inclusion criteria for problems which are common in general/family practice, and which require inclusion criteria if they are to be coded consistently.

Another major advantage of this framework is that employing minimal inclusion criteria results in coding procedures which are easy to learn and apply in the real world of general/family practice. This will reduce the magnitude of the problem of intercoder variation.

Using inclusion criteria

Inclusion criteria SHOULD NOT be used when recording reasons for encounter, since these should be coded in terms of what the doctor understands the patient to say, irrespective of whether or not the patient is 'correct'.

Inclusion criteria SHOULD be used when coding the diagnoses or problems the doctor manages. Even when the problem has to be coded only as a symptom or complaint, some guidance may be needed in order to select the most appropriate code. For example, feeling faint (N17) is not coded in the same rubric as actual fainting (A06); and abdominal pain may be generalized (D01), epigastric (D02), or localized in other regions (D06). The options need to be clear to users so that the most appropriate alternative is used.

Applying the criteria at different stages of the problem

The inclusion criteria are primarily designed to code the early presentation of a problem. If the problem is to be coded during a later encounter (after its modification by time or therapy) the coder should consider the historical information (e.g. blood pressure may well be normal at later consultations in a patient with hypertension receiving therapy but the condition would still be coded as hypertension).

Disadvantages of the system

Clearly, this system of inclusion criteria is not without hazard. In order to improve the accuracy and reliability of statistics from general/family practice, hard edges have been put to diagnostic concepts, many of which seem, in reality, to have blurred borders.

Although sharp borders may not be needed for therapy or management, accurate data are needed for purposes of research. The use of hard-edged inclusion criteria may increase the content of residual less specific rubrics, but this is preferred to making most rubrics non-specific. For coding problems which do not fully meet the given criteria, less specific alternatives are suggested following 'Consider:'. These suggestions are in addition to those items which are listed as exclusions in the rubric.

Some possible misconceptions

It is important that the reader clearly understand several things which the criteria are NOT intended to do.

1. *They do not serve as a guide to diagnosis.* The primary purpose of the classification is to reduce chances of miscoding after a diagnosis has been made, and not to eliminate the possibility of diagnostic error. The assumption is that the user will have considered the differential diagnosis prior to the time of coding. In most cases good practice of medicine requires far more information than is given in the inclusion criteria to make accurate diagnoses.
2. *They do not set standards for care.* Although information derived from the use of the classification may change medical concepts and ultimately impact on standards of care, these inclusion criteria are intended solely to improve the quality of data recording.
3. *They do not act as a guide for therapy.* The criteria given for inclusion or exclusion for a condition do not necessarily relate to the criteria for use of various therapies. For example, the practitioner may well decide that therapy for migraine is indicated in a patient whose findings were insufficient to fulfil the criteria listed under that diagnostic title, and whose condition is coded as 'headache'.

Sources

The Committee felt no compulsion to devise new definitions and based inclusion criteria on existing ones, if appropriate for the objectives given above. In fact, few existing definitions did meet those requirements because most had been prepared for research projects rather than for clinical practice and so tended to be rather cumbersome. However, the inclusion criteria included here are compatible with most standard definitions of diseases.

If someone else's work has been used inadvertently without acknowledgement, apologies are given: imitation is the sincerest form of flattery.

7 Severity of illness coding

Development of severity of illness coding

Since 1993 the WONCA Classification Committee has been developing the Duke Severity of Illness Checklist (DUSOI) system[26] for international use. The WONCA Severity of Illness Field Trial (WONCA-SIFT) was conducted to test the system in 16 countries.[27] The committee recognized that a method is needed to enable doctors to code not only the name of each health problem, but also the level of severity of each problem. This is applicable to problems whether in respect of episode of care, or for each encounter (see Fig. 2).

The ICPC is now unique among international classification systems in that it can be used to classify health problems by their level of severity in the individual patient with the health problem. The severity coding system, the Duke/WONCA Severity of Illness Checklist (DUSOI/WONCA), is an extension that enables the physician or other health worker not only to give the problem a standardized title and classification code, but also a standardized severity code that indicates which patients with the same health problem have the more or less severe problem. Since the severity parameters and criteria of the system are generic, not health problem specific, they can be applied to any health problem. This generic quality also allows comparison of the severity of different health problems based upon the same standards for assessment. The system is feasible for use by family/general practitioners in the clinical setting as demonstrated in the WONCA-SIFT field trial.[27]

Coding severity of illness

The DUSOI/WONCA severity of illness coding system allows ICPC to be used to classify health problems in terms of severity. To code severity, the health care provider identifies each problem at the time of patient encounter and determines how severe each problem is for that particular patient at that particular time. Severity is based upon the following four generic parameters:

1. *Symptoms* during the past week.
2. *Complications* during the past week.
3. *Prognosis* during the next six months if no treatment were to be given for the health problem.
4. *Treatability*, or the need for treatment and the expected response to treatment by this patient.

An example of a completed form is shown in Fig. 4, in which the provider, John Smith, has listed the current health problems which he addressed during the encounter for

DUKE/WONCA SEVERITY OF ILLNESS CHECKLIST: **DUSOI/WONCA***   Patient: Mary Jones

Birthdate: Nov. 6, 1925   Female: ✓   Male: Provider: John Smith   Date of Encounter: Oct. 5, 1995

Health Problems (Addressed during this encounter)	Raw Scores (Enter 0-4)**				Total Raw Score (0-16)	Severity Code*** (0-4)	ICPC Code
	Symptoms	Complications	Prognosis	Treatability			
EXAMPLE: Gout	3	1	3	2	9	3	T92:3
1. Ischaemic Heart Disease without Angina	2	0	4	2	8	2	K76:2
2. Diabetes Mellitus	0	0	2	2	4	1	T90:1
3. Acute Bronchitis	3	0	2	2	7	2	R78:2
4.							
5.							
6.							

(Use additional pages if more than six health problems.)

**RAW SCORES

	None	Questionable	Mild	Moderate	Major
1. Symptoms (past week):	0	1	2	3	4
2. Complications (past week):	0	1	2	3	4

3. Prognosis (next 6 months, without treatment):			Disability			Threat to Life
	None	Mild	Moderate	Major		
	0	1	2	3		4

	Need for Treatment			Expected Response to Treatment		
	No	Questionable	IF YES →→	Good	Questionable	Poor
4. Treatability:	0	1		2	3	4

*** SEVERITY CODES

Total Raw Score		Severity Code		Severity
0	=	0		None
1-4	=	1		Mild
5-8	=	2		Intermediate
9-12	=	3		Moderate
13-16	=	4		Maximum

Fig. 4. Duke/WONCA severity of illness checklist: DUSOI/WONCA.

*Copyright © 1996, Department of Community and Family Medicine, Duke University Medical Center, Curham, NC, USA

patient Mary Jones on 5 October 1995. Gout is printed on all forms as an example; it does not apply to this patient. If patient Jones had had gout, the provider would have listed gout again and scored its severity according to its specific effects on Mary Jones. Actually, at this encounter this patient had ischaemic heart disease without angina, diabetes mellitus, and acute bronchitis.

Raw scores

The raw severity scores that are possible for each of the four severity parameters are shown in the large box at the bottom of the DUSOI/WONCA form. In the example of ischaemic heart disease without angina (K76) in Fig. 4, the severity of *symptoms* was rated '2' on a scale of 0 to 4, because the patient was considered to have mild symptoms at that time. Severity in terms of complications was rated '0' because no complications for ischaemic heart disease were evident clinically. For DUSOI/WONCA ratings, the definition of a complication is 'a health problem which is secondary to another health problem, but which is not listed and rated as a separate problem'. If a *complication* is recorded on the form as a separate health problem, the effects of this separately recorded complication should not be included in the severity rating of the health problem of origin, in order to avoid assigning double weight to a complication in the scoring. *Prognosis* for ischaemic heart disease with angina in Fig. 4 was scored '4' because the provider made a clinical judgment that this patient would be expected to die during the next six months following the encounter if no treatment were given, thereby allowing the heart disease to have full effect on the untreated patient. If Dr Smith had predicted that Mary Jones would not die without treatment, but rather would experience major disability, then a rating of '3' for prognosis would have been appropriate. Disability is defined as 'any limitation of a person's ability to function in everyday life'. Major disability (raw score 3) is defined as 'much restriction of usual activity and much care needed from others'. Mild disability (raw score 1) is defined as 'little restriction of usual activities', and moderate disability (raw score 2) is defined as 'much restriction of usual activity but little care needed from others'. *Treatability* was rated '2' in the example because the provider decided that this particular patient needed treatment and would be expected to have a good response to that treatment.

Severity codes

To determine the single-digit DUSOI/WONCA severity code, the raw scores for each health problem are summed, and the total raw score is converted to a severity code using the conversion table in the small box at the bottom of the form. In the example of ischaemic heart disease without angina in Fig. 4, the total raw score = 8(2 + 0 + 4 + 2), and the severity code = 2. (The conversion table shows that raw scores of 5 to 8 = a severity code of 2.) The severity code of 2 indicates that ischaemic heart disease without angina in this particular patient at this particular encounter is of intermediate severity, on a scale of 0 to 4 from 'none' to 'maximum' severity.

The severity code can be added to the problem code as an extension, using ':' as the link, a convention which distinguishes the severity extension from other extensions which may be used. Hence the code for the ischaemic heart disease without angina in Fig. 4 is K76:2.

Results of the severity of illness field trial (WOIMCA-SIFT)

The international study was conducted during a two-year period (1993–5) to test the reliability, feasibility, and potential clinical usefulness of the DUSOI/WONCA. Initially 47 general/family practitioners from 16 different countries participated. Of these, 22 practitioners from 9 countries (Belgium, Germany, Hong Kong, Israel, Japan, The Netherlands, Spain, The United Kingdom, and The United States) completed data collection.[27]

The 22 practitioners performed DUSOI/WONCA ratings on 1191 patients. The study group had a mean age of 59.2 years; 59.6% were females; and they had a total of 2488 health problems. Reliability of the DUSOI/WONCA was estimated from ratings on a series of standardized health problems. The intraclass correlation coefficient (ICC)[28] for interrater reliability was 0.45 and the ICC for intrarater reliability ranged from a low of 0.39 for the social problem of partner being ill (ICPC code Z14), to 0.78 for obesity (ICPC code T82) and 0.68 for anxiety (ICPC code P74). Feasibility for use in practice was good, as indicated by an average of only 1.9 minutes required to rate the DUSOI/WONCA on each patient (ranging from less than 1 to 10 minutes). The physicians experienced no difficulty in using the system in 71.1% of patients. They found it quite useful in 14.7% of patients, somewhat useful in 53.6%, and of no use in 31.7%. Usefulness was higher in patients with higher severity of illness scores.

The mean DUSOI/WONCA severity score for all 2488 health problems was 39.1 (scale = 0–100 from lowest to highest severity), and the problems were distributed among the five severity classification codes as follows: Code 0 (no severity) = 1.6%, Code 1 (mild severity) = 29.9%, Code 2 (intermediate severity) = 45.9%, Code 3 (moderate severity) = 19.3%, and Code 4 (maximum severity) = 3.3%. Wide variations in severity were shown, both between different diagnoses and within each diagnosis. For example, mean severity for respiratory health problems varied between 26.4 for upper respiratory infection (URI, ICPC code R74) to 53.2 for chronic obstructive pulmonary disease (COPD, ICPC code R95). For URI, the frequency of severity codes ranged from 61.1% for Code 1 to 0% for Code 4, in contrast to COPD with the range from 8.4% for Code 1 to 10.6% with Code 4.

When surveyed at the end of the field trial concerning their future anticipated personal use of the DUSOI/WONCA, 41.2% of the 22 participants reported they might use it in patient care, 71.2% might use it in research, 43.8% in teaching, and 52.9% in practice management.

It was concluded that the DUSOI/WONCA is feasible and potentially useful clinically in family/general practice.[27] Although the practitioners were not queried about the usefulness of the system for disease severity classification, the empirical findings of the field trial indicate that it is well suited for this purpose.

8 Functional status assessment: the COOP/WONCA charts

In 1987 the WONCA Classification Committee began to develop a way of classifying and recording the overall functional status of the patient as distinct from the status of severity of their health problem(s).[29] Over a number of years this work, later conducted in cooperation with the WONCA Research Committee, resulted in production of the COOP/WONCA Functional Status Assessment Charts.[30,31]

Functional status is a measure of an individual's overall well-being. It is one of the set of global measures of health status, which also include assessments of clinical status and quality of life. The International Glossary for General/Family Practice defines functional status as 'the ability of a person to perform and adapt to his/her environment, measured both objectively and subjectively over a stated period of time'.[19] Implicit in any definition of functional status is the importance of factors other than disease in the health of patients. As the complexity and chronicity of medical problems increase, general/family practitioners will become more reliant on indicators of functioning as well as disease status to monitor their interventions and measure health outcomes.

Functional status relates to the patient, not to the health problem, disease, or episode of care. It thus relates less directly to the ICPC codes than does severity of illness. However, its importance in general/family practice warrants its inclusion in this book.

For some time general practitioners have recognized the integral importance of health promotion and the measurement of functional status in consultations. These measurements are particularly important in dealing with ageing and those with chronic problems. The addition of functional status measures to the recording of reason for encounter, diagnosis, and therapeutic interventions is a logical step for the process of classification in general/family practice.

Instruments for measuring functional status

One of the first instruments to be recognized by WONCA as a reliable and practical measure of functional status in the family practice setting was the Dartmouth COOP Functional Assessment Charts.[32] These charts were modified by the classification committee and promoted for use in conjunction with ICPC. The revised charts are known as the COOP/WONCA charts.

The COOP/WONCA charts, whilst specifically developed for general/family practice, are not the only instruments available for assessing functional status. There are a plethora of indicators currently available. Several have been used in general practice settings.

The Medical Outcomes Trust Short Form 36-item inventory and derivatives of this instrument have been widely used in primary care settings. Similarly, the Duke Health Profile has been used successfully in North American settings.[33] In Europe, several other instruments have been used. The Sickness Impact Profile (SIP) and the Nottingham Health Profile (NHP) are the two most widely cited. Some of these instruments were designed for research not clinical purposes, (e.g. the Sickness Impact Profile[34]).

To date, the COOP/WONCA charts have been tested most extensively in general/family practice settings.[35] Internationally, they have been found to have good face validity and clinical utility in general practice.[36] General practitioners have found the charts easy to use within the consultation and helpful as measures of overall patient status and as outcomes of care.

With any measure of functional status, cultural and context issues need to be explored. Some studies of the charts have suggested that they do not exhibit cross-cultural stability. As a research instrument the test-retest reliability will always be an issue for indicators that are global and influenced by so many variables. Several studies have looked at these issues. Standardization of test conditions and assessment of intrarater reliability may improve the results for research projects.

COOP/WONCA charts

The current form of the COOP/WONCA charts was determined through extensive testing in general/family practice settings. There are now six charts: physical fitness; feelings; daily activities; social activities; change in health; and overall health. An example of the Daily Activities Chart is shown in Fig. 5. Additional charts for pain and sleep are under development.

Each chart consists of a lead sentence with five options for response. Pictorial depictions of the five possible responses accompany the text. These drawings have enhanced the applicability of these charts in settings where there is variability of literacy amongst the general practice patient population.

To date the charts have been published in the following languages: Chinese, Danish, Dutch, Finnish, French, German, Hebrew, Italian, Japanese, Korean, Norwegian, Portuguese, Spanish (Catalan, Castilian, and Callego), Slovak, Swedish, and Urdu.[31]

Use of the charts

The charts can be used independently or in groups. When more than one chart is used it is recommended that they are administered in the following order: physical fitness, feelings, daily activities, social activities, change in health, overall health. The preferred method of use of these charts is self-administration. However, one study has shown a correlation between self-assessment and provider assessment.[31] The average time for completion of the six charts is less than five minutes.

When the charts are used in new cultural settings, it is important to establish that the concepts measured are appropriate and specific to that environment. Appropriate translation is the first step.

Daily activities

During the past 2 weeks...
How much difficulty have you had doing our usual activities or
tasks, both inside and outside the house, because of your physical
and emotional health?

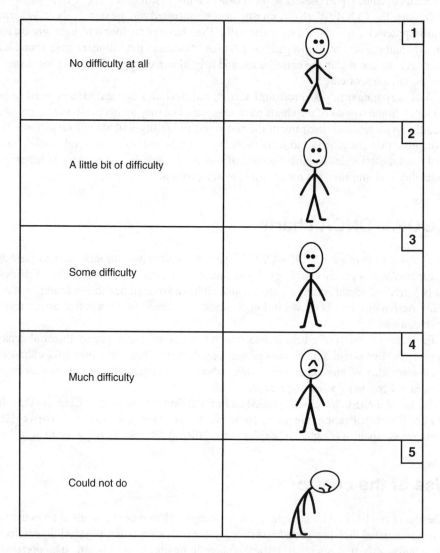

No difficulty at all		1
A little bit of difficulty		2
Some difficulty		3
Much difficulty		4
Could not do		5

Fig. 5. COOP/WONCA Functional Health Status Chart: daily activities.

Measuring functional health status with the COOP/WONCA Charts: a Manual,[31] provides further information about the development and use of the charts, how to translate the charts, and a contact list for further assistance, including authors of the various translations.

Relationship between ICPC and the COOP/WONCA charts

Together with ICPC the COOP/WONCA charts can be used to explore the relationship between functionality and health problems. For example, Rubric 28 of Component 1 (symptoms and complaints) of all chapters of ICPC refers to limited function and disabilities. Functional status could be coded in this component with the addition of an extra digit. However, since functional status relates to the patient as a whole and not to the health problem, the relationship becomes difficult to interpret when there is more than one active problem, because comorbidity complicates the interpretation. For example, hypertension and diabetes in one patient can both impact on functional status, but their relative importance and effects cannot be determined from routine recording. Even with only one problem, functional status measures go beyond assessing problem status and therefore their relationship to a particular ICPC code may not be straightforward.

9 References

1. International classification of diseases (9th revision). Geneva, World Health Organization, 1977.
2. International Statistical Classification of Diseases and Related Health Problems (10th revision). Geneva, World Health Organization, 1992.
3. International Classification of Health Problems in Primary Care (ICHPPC). Chicago, World Organization National Colleges, Academies and Academic Associations of General Practitioners/Family Physicians (WONCA)/American Hospital Association (AHA), 1975.
4. ICHPPC-2 (International Classification of Health Problems in Primary Care). Oxford, Oxford University Press, 1979.
5. ICHPPC-2-Defined: International Classification of Health Problems in Primary Care, 3rd edition. Oxford, Oxford University Press, 1983.
6. Report of the International Conference on Primary Care, Alma Ata, USSR, 6–12 September 1978; WHO/Alma Ata/78.10.
7. Meads S. The WHO Reason for Encounter classification. *WHO Chronicle* 1983; **37**(5): 159–162.
8. Lamberts H, Meads S, and Wood M. Classification of reasons why persons seek primary care: pilot study of a new system. *Public Health Rep.* 1984; **99**: 597–605.
9. Lamberts H, Meads S, and Wood M. Results of the international field trial with the Reason for Encounter Classification (RFEC). *Med. Sociale Preventive* 1985; **30**: 80–87.
10. Working party to develop a classification of the 'Reasons for Contact with Primary Health Care Services'. Report to the World Health Organization, Geneva, Switzerland, 1981.
11. Wood M. Family medicine classification systems in evolution. *J. Fam. Pract.* 1981; **12**: 199–200.
12. Lamberts H, Meads S, and Wood M. Results of the field trial with the Reason for Encounter Classification (RFEC). In: Cote R A, Protti A J, and Schemer J R (ed.) Role of Informatics in Health Data Coding and Classification Systems. Amsterdam, Elsevier/JFIP-JMIA, 1985.
13. Bentsen B G. International Classification of Primary Care. *Scand. J. Prim. Health Care* 1986; **4**: 43–56.
14. Lamberts H, Wood M, Hofmans-Okkes I (ed.). The International Classification of Primary Care in the European Community: with Multi-Language Layer. Oxford, Oxford University Press, 1993.
15. Lamberts H and Wood M (ed.). ICPC: International Classification of Primary Care. Oxford, Oxford University Press, 1987.
16. Bridges-Webb C, Britt H, Miles D A, Neary S, Charles J, and Traynor V. Morbidity and treatment in general practice in Australia 1990–1991. *Med. J. Aust.* 1992; **157**, Suppl. 19 Oct: S1–S56.

17. Hofmans-Okkes I M and Lamberts H. The International Classification of Primary Care (ICPC): new applications in research and computer based patient records in family practice. *Fam. Pract.* 1996; **13**: 294–302.

18. Wood M, Lamberts H, Meijer J S, and Hofmans-Okkes I M. The conversion between ICPC and ICD-10: requirements for a family of classification systems in the next decade. In: Lamberts H, Wood M, and Hofman-Okkes I (ed.) The International Classification of Primary Care in the European Community: with Multi-Language Layer. Oxford, Oxford University Press, 1993: 18–24.

19. Bentzen N (ed.). An international glossary for general/family practice. *Fam. Pract.* 1995; **12**: 341–369.

20. Jamoulle M and Roland M. Classification Internationale des Soins Primaires (traduction francaise de l'ICPC). Edition Alexandre Lacassagne, Lyon, 1992.

21. Jamoulle M and Roland M. Approches taxonomiques en medicine de famille, assorties d'une terminologie medicale normalisee et classifiee a usage informatique en soins de sante primaires. CARE Editions, Brussels, 2 vol., 1996.

22. Donaldson M S, Yordy K D, Lohr K N, and Vanselow N A (ed.). Primary care: America's health in a new era. Washington DC, National Academy Press, 1996.

23. Hofmans-Okkes I M. An international study into the concept and validity of the 'reason for encounter'. In: Lamberts H, Wood M, and Hofmans-Okkes I M (ed.) The International Classification of Primary Care in the European Community. Oxford, Oxford University Press, 1993: 34–44.

24. Nylenna, M. Why do our patients see us? A study of reasons for encounter in general practice. *Scand. J. Prim. Health Care* 1985; **3**: 155–162.

25. International Classification of Process in Primary Care (IC-Process-PC). Oxford, Oxford University Press, 1986.

26. Parkerson G R Jr, Broadhead W E, and Tse C-K J. The Duke Severity of Illness Checklist (DUSOI) for measurement of severity and comorbidity. *J. Clin. Epidemiol.* 1993; **46**: 379–393.

27. Parkerson G R Jr, Bridges-Webb C, Gervas J, Hofmans-Okkes I, Lamberts H, Froom J, Fischer G, Meyboom-de Jong B, Klinkman M, and Maeseneer J. Classification of severity of health problems in family/general practice: an international field trial. *Fam. Pract.* 1996; **13**: 303–309.

28. Shrout P E and Fleiss J L. Intraclass correlations: uses in assessing rater reliability. *Psychol. Bull.* 1979; **86**: 420–428.

29. WONCA Classification Committee. Functional status in primary care. New York, Springer, 1990.

30. Scholten J H G and van Weel C. Functional Status Assessment in Family Practice. MEDITekst CIP-Gegevens Koninklikje Bibliotheek, The Hague, 1992.

31. van Weel C, Konig-Zahn C, Touw-Otten F W M M, van Duijn N P, and Meyboom-de Jong B. Measuring functional health status with the COOPAVONCA Charts: a manual. CIP-Gegevens Koninklijke Bibiliotheek, The Hague, 1995.

32. Nelson E C, Wasson J, Kirk J, *et al.* Assessment of function in routine clinical practice. Description of the COOP chart method and preliminary findings. *J. Chron. Dis.* 1987; **40** (Suppl. 1): 55s–64s.

33. Parkerson G R Jr, Broadhead W E, and Tse C-K J. The Duke Health Profile, a 17-item measure of health and dysfunction. *Med. Care* 1990; **28**: 1056–1072.

34. Bergner M, Bobbin R A, Carter W B, *et al*. The Sickness Impact Profile. Conceptual formulation and methodology for the development of a health status measure. *Int. J. Health Serv.* 1976; **6**: 393.

35. Hutchinson A, Bentzen N, Konig-Zahn C (eds.). Cross cultural health outcome assessment: a user's guide. *European Research Group on Health Outcomes* (ERGHO), 1997; 1–184.

36. Bentsen B, Natvig B, Winnem M. Assessment of own functional capacity. COOP-WONCA charts in clinical work and research (in Norwegian, English summary). *Tiddsk. Nor. Laegeforen.* 1997; **117**: 1790–93.

10 International Classification of Primary Care-2-Revised: tabular list

This tabular list consists of details of all the rubrics in ICPC-2-Revised and is a major revision of the tabular list of the ICPC-2, published in 1998.[1] It includes the revisions of ICPC-2 in 2000[2] and 2002[3] and more recent unpublished revisions decided upon in WICC meetings in 2003 and 2004. The editors of this revision are Inge Okkes, Henk Becker, Sibo Oskam, and Henk Lamberts of the Department of Family Practice, University of Amsterdam, The Netherlands.

Chapter 11 includes the revised conversion with ICD-10.

The process components 2–6, which are standard in all chapters, are set out first, followed by components 1 and 7 in which each rubric is specific in each chapter.

1. WONCA International Classification Committee. International Classification for Primary Care, 2nd edn. (ICPC-2). Oxford, Oxford University Press, 1998.
2. Okkes I M, Jamoulle M, Lamberts H, Bentzen N. ICPC-2-E. The electronic version of ICPC-2. Differences with the printed version and the consequences. *Fam. Pract.* 2000; **17**: 101–106.
3. Okkes I M, Becker H W, Bernstein R M, Lamberts H. The March 2002 update of the electronic version of ICPC-2. A step forward to the use of ICD-10 as a nomenclature and a terminology for ICPC-2. *Fam. Pract.* 2002; **19**: 543–546.

Standard process components of ICPC: components 2–6

The dash (—) shown in first position must be replaced with the appropriate alpha code for each chapter.

Component 2—Diagnostic and preventive procedures

—30 Medical examination/health evaluation—complete
—31 Medical examination/health evaluation—partial
—32 Sensitivity test
—33 Microbiological/immunological test
—34 Blood test
—35 Urine test

—36   Faeces test
—37   Histological/exfoliative cytology
—38   Other laboratory test NEC
—39   Physical function test
—40   Diagnostic endoscopy
—41   Diagnostic radiology/imaging
—42   Electrical tracings
—43   Other diagnostic procedures
—44   Preventive immunizations/medications
—45   Observation/health education/advice/diet
—46   Consultation with primary care provider
—47   Consultation with specialist
—48   Clarification/discussion of patient's RFE/demand
—49   Other preventive procedures

Component 3—Medication, treatment, therapeutic procedures

—50   Medication-prescription/request/renewal/injection
—51   Incision/drainage/flushing/aspiration/removal body fluid (*excl.* catheterization—53)
—52   Excision/removal tissue/biopsy/destruction/debridement/cauterization
—53   Instrumentation/catheterization/intubation/dilation
—54   Repair/fixation–suture/cast/prosthetic device (apply/remove)
—55   Local injection/infiltration
—56   Dressing/pressure/compression/tamponade
—57   Physical medicine/rehabilitation
—58   Therapeutic counselling/listening
—59   Other therapeutic procedures/minor surgery, NEC

Component 4—Results

—60   Results tests/procedures
—61   Results examination/test/record/letter from other provider

Component 5—Administrative

—62   Administrative procedure

Component 6—Referrals and other reasons for encounter

—63   Follow-up encounter unspecified
—64   Encounter/problem initiated by provider
—65   Encounter/problem initiated by other than patient/provider
—66   Referral to other provider/nurse/therapist/social worker (*excl.* medical)
—67   Referral to physician/specialist/clinic/hospital

—68   Other referrals NEC
—69   Other reason for encounter NEC

Layout of rubrics in components 1 and 7

Rubrics are set out in the following format:

Code	Title	*ICD-10 code(s)*
incl:	*terms included*	
excl:	*terms excluded, with their ICPC codes*	
criteria:	*criteria for inclusion in this rubric*	
consider:	*rubrics to be considered if the criteria are not met*	

Example:

A73 Malaria   *B50 to B54*

incl:	complications of malaria
criteria:	intermittent fever with chills and rigors in a resident of, or recent visitor to, a malarial region; or demonstration of malarial parasite forms in the peripheral blood
consider:	fever A03

Summary of main changes to Components 1 and 7 from ICPC-1 to ICPC-2

Only major changes are listed here: additions, change in meaning of the rubric, or transfer or deletion of a rubric. There are many other changes of detail to the titles of the rubrics that do not change the meaning, and are not listed here.

CODE	TITLE ICPC-1 (some abbreviated)	TITLE ICPC-2
A05	GENERAL DETERIORATION	FEELING ILL
A11	(omitted by mistake from ICPC)	CHEST PAIN NOS
A12	ALLERGY/ALLERGIC REACTION	(transferred to A92)
A13	CONCERN ABOUT DRUG REACTION	CONCERN/FEAR ABOUT TREATMENT
A14	INFANTILE COLIC	(deleted, included in D01)
A15	EXCESSIVE CRYING INFANT	(deleted, included in A16)
A17	OTHER GEN SYMPT INFANT	(deleted, included in A16)
A18	(new rubric in ICPC-2)	CONCERN ABOUT APPEARANCE
A21	(new rubric in ICPC-2)	RISK FACTOR FOR MALIGNANCY

A23	(new rubric in ICPC-2)	RISK FACTOR NOS
A92	TOXOPLASMOSIS	ALLERGY/ALLERGIC
	(deleted, included with A78)	REACTION NOS
		(transferred from A12)
A98	(new rubric in ICPC-2)	HEALTH MAINTENANCE/
		PREVENTIVE MEDICINE
B03	OTHER SYMPT	(deleted, included in B02)
	LYMPH GLANDS	
B85	UNEXPLAINED ABNORMAL	(deleted, included in A91)
	BLOOD TEST	
B86	OTHER HAEMATOLOGICAL	(deleted, included in B99)
	ABNORMALITY	
D07	(new rubric in ICPC-2)	DYSPEPSIA/INDIGESTION
D22	WORMS/PINWORMS/OTHER	(transferred to D96)
	PARASITES	
D23	(transferred from D96)	HEPATOMEGALY
D96	HEPATOMEGALY	(transferred to D23)
D96	(changed rubric in ICPC-2)	WORMS/OTHER PARASITES
K22	(new rubric in ICPC-2)	RISK FACTOR FOR CAR-
		DIOVASCULAR DISEASE
K74	ANGINA PECTORIS	ISCHAEMIC HEART
		DISEASE WITH ANGINA
K76	OTHER AND CHRONIC	ISCHAEMIC HEART
	ISCHAEMIC HEART	DISEASE, NO ANGINA
K80	ECTOPIC BEATS, ALL TYPES	CARDIAC ARRHYTHMIA NOS
K81	HEART MURMER, NOS	HEART/ARTERIAL
		MURMER, NOS
K91	ATHEROSCLEROSIS	(included with K92 in ICPC-2)
	(EXCL. HEART/BRAIN)	
K91	(altered rubric in ICPC-2)	CEREBROVASCULAR DISEASE
K92	OTHER ARTERIAL	ATHEROSCLEROSIS/
	OBSTRUCTION/PER	PERIPH VASC DIS
L05	FLANK SYMPTOMS/	FLANK/AXILLA
	COMPLAINTS	SYMPTOMS/COMPLAINTS
L06	AXILLA SYMPTOMS/	(deleted, included in L05)
	COMPLAINTS	
L71	NEOPLASMS	MALIGNANT NEOPLASM
L83	SYNDROMES RELATED	NECK SYNDROME
	TO CERVICAL SPINE	
L84	OSTEOARTHRITIS OF	BACK SYNDROME
	SPINE (ANY R)	WITHOUT RADIATION
L86	LUMBAR DISC LESION,	DISC LESION/BACK PAIN
	BACK PAIN	WITH RADIATION
L87	GANGLION JOINT/	BURSITIS/TENDONITIS/
	TENDON	SYNOVITIS NOS

L97	CHRONIC INTERNAL KNEE DERANGEM (included with L99 IN ICPC-2)	NEOPLASM, BENIGN/ UNCERTAIN (split from L71 in ICPC-2)
N02	TENSION HEADACHE	(transferred to N95)
N08	(new rubric in ICPC-2)	ABNORMAL INVOLUNTARY MOVEMENTS (split from N06)
N80	OTHER HEAD INJURY WITHOUT SKULL FRACTURE	HEAD INJURY, OTHER
N95	(new rubric in ICPC-2)	TENSION HEADACHE (transferred from N02)
P21	OVERACTIVE CHILD, HYPERKINETIC	(transferred to P81)
P75	HYSTERICAL/ HYPOCHONDRIACAL DIS	SOMATIZATION DISORDER
P81	(new rubric in ICPC-2)	HYPERKINETIC DISORDER (transferred from P21)
P82	(new rubric in ICPC-2)	POST-TRAUMATIC STRESS DISORDER (split from P02)
P86	(new rubric in ICPC-2)	ANOREXIA NERVOSA, BULIMIA (transferred from T06)
R22	SYMPTOM/COMPLAINT TONSILS	(deleted, included in R21)
R70	TUBERCULOSIS	(deleted, included in A70)
R72	STREP-THROAT/SCARLET FEVER	STREP THROAT (scarlet fever included in A78)
R79	(new rubric in ICPC-2)	CHRONIC BRONCHITIS (transferred from R91)
R80	INFLUENZA WITHOUT PNEUMONIA	INFLUENZA
R82	PLEURISY	PLEURISY/PLEURAL EFFUSION (includes pleural effusion from R93)
R91	CHRONIC BRONCHITIS	(transferred to R79)
R92	(new rubric in ICPC-2)	NEOPLASM RESPIRATORY, UNCERTAIN NATURE
R93	PLEURAL EFFUSION	(deleted, included in R82)
S11	OTHER LOCALIZED SKIN INFECTION	WOUNDINFECTION, POST-TRAUMATIC
S79	OTHER BENIGN NEOPLASMS OF SKIN	NEOPLASM SKIN, BENIGN/UNCERTAIN
S80	OTHER UNSPECIFIED NEOPLASM SKIN	SOLAR KERATOSIS/SUNBURN
T06	ANOREXIA NERVOSA W/WO BULIMIA	(transferred to P82)
T15	THYROID LUMP/MASS	(deleted, included in T81)
T88	RENAL GLYCOSURIA	(deleted, included in T99)

T89	(new rubric in ICPC-2)	DIABETES, INSULIN DEPENDENT
T90	DIABETES MELLITUS	DIABETES, NON-INSULIN DEPENDENT
U08	(new rubric in ICPC-2)	URINARY RETENTION
W20	OTHER SYMPTOMS/COMPLAINTS OF BREAST	(deleted, included in W19)
W21	(new rubric in ICPC-2)	CONCERN ABOUT BODY IMAGE IN PREGNANCY
W77	OTHER NON-OBSTETRICAL CONDITION	(deleted)
W85	(new rubric in ICPC-2)	GESTATIONAL DIABETES
X22	(new rubric in ICPC-2)	CONCERN ABOUT BREAST APPEARANCE
X92	(new rubric in ICPC-2)	CHLAMYDIA INFECTION, GENITAL

A General and unspecified

Component 1—Symptoms and complaints

Note: In this classification general or multiple refers to three or more body sites or systems. Conditions affecting one or two sites should be coded to the appropriate sites.

A01 Pain, general/multiple sites   *R52*

incl: chronic general pain, multiple aches

A02 Chills   *R68.8*

incl: rigors, shivers
excl: fever A03

A03 Fever   *R50*

incl: pyrexia
excl: fever with rash A76; heat exhaustion/stroke A88

A04 Weakness/tiredness, general   *G93.3, R53*

incl: chronic fatigue syndrome, exhaustion, fatigue, lassitude, lethargy, postviral fatigue
excl: malaise/feeling ill A05; drowsy A29; heat exhaustion A88; jetlag A88; somnolence P06

A05 Feeling ill
R53

incl: malaise
excl: senescence/senility P05; cachexia T08; malnutrition T91

A06 Fainting/syncope
R55

incl: blackout, collapse, vasovagal attack
excl: coma A07; feeling faint/giddiness/dizziness N17

A07 Coma
R40

incl: stupor
excl: syncope A06

A08 Swelling
R68.8

incl: lump, mass NOS
excl: enlarged lymph gland B02; oedema K07; swelling joint L20; swelling breast X19, Y16

A09 Sweating problem
R61

incl: hyperhidrosis, night sweats, perspiration problem
excl: sweat gland disease S92

A10 Bleeding/haemorrhage NOS
R58

A11 Chest pain NOS
R07.4

excl: pain attributed to heart K01; pain attributed to chest wall L04; pain attributed to respiratory system R01

A13 Concern about/fear of medical treatment
Z71.1

incl: concern about/fear of the consequences of drug/medical treatment
excl: adverse effect of drug A85; complication of medical/surgical treatment A87

A16 Irritable infant
R68.1

incl: excessively crying/restless infant
excl: infantile colic D01; restless child/adult P04

A18 Concern about appearance
R46.8

excl: concern about appearance of ears H15; concern about appearance in pregnancy W21; concern about appearance of breasts X22

A20 Euthanasia request/discussion   *Z71.8*

A21 Risk factor for malignancy   *Z80, Z85*

incl: personal/family history of malignancy, past treatment, other risk factor for malignancy

A23 Risk factor NOS

Z20, Z28, Z72.0 to Z72.5, Z73.2, Z81, Z82.0 to Z82.2, Z82.5 to Z82.8, Z83, Z84, Z86.0 to Z86.6, Z87, Z88, Z91, Z92

incl: contact with infectious disease, personal/family history, previous episode, other risk factor for other disease
excl: risk factor for malignancy A21; risk factor for cardiovascular disease K22

A25 Fear of death/dying   *Z71.1*

A26 Fear of cancer NOS   *Z71.1*

excl: if the patient has cancer, code the disease
criteria: concern about/fear of cancer not related to a specific chapter in a patient without the disease/until the diagnosis is proven

A27 Fear of other disease NOS   *Z71.1*

excl: fear of cancer NOS A26; if the patient has the disease, code the disease
criteria: concern about/fear of an other disease not related to a specific chapter in a patient without the disease/until the diagnosis is proven

A28 Limited function/disability NOS

Z73.6, Z74, Z99.0, Z99.3, Z99.8, Z99.9

excl: falls A29
criteria: limitation of function/disability not related to a problem in any other chapter
Note: The COOP/WONCA Charts are suitable for documenting the patient's functional status (see Chapter 8).

A29 General symptom/complaint, other   *R26.8, R68.0, R68.8*

incl: clumsiness, drowsy, falls

Component 7—diagnoses/diseases

A70 Tuberculosis   *A15 to A19, B90, N74.0, N74.1*

incl: tuberculosis infection of any body site, late effect of tuberculosis
criteria: conversion to a positive tuberculin skin test; or demonstration of *Mycobacterium tuberculosis* on microscopy or culture; or characteristic

(cont.)

chest X-ray appearance; or characteristic histological appearance on biopsy

consider: fever A03; cough R05

A71 Measles   *B05*

incl: complications of measles
criteria: prodrome with injected conjunctivae, fever, and cough; plus white specks on a red base in the mucous membranes of the cheek (Koplik's spots), or confluent maculopapular eruption spreading over the face and body, or an atypical exanthem in a partially immune person during an epidemic of measles; or serological evidence of acute measles
consider: fever A03; other viral exanthem A76; generalized rash S07

A72 Chickenpox   *B01*

incl: complications of chickenpox
excl: herpes zoster S70
criteria: a vesicular exanthem that appears in successive crops, with the lesions evolving rapidly from superficial papules to vesicles and eventually to scabs
consider: fever A03; other viral exanthem A76; generalized rash S07

A73 Malaria   *B50 to B54*

incl: complications of malaria
criteria: intermittent fever with chills and rigors in resident of/recent visitor to a malarial region; or demonstration of malarial parasite forms in the peripheral blood
consider: fever A03

A74 Rubella   *B06*

incl: complications of rubella
excl: congenital rubella A94; roseola infantum A76
criteria: an acute exanthem with enlarged lymph nodes, most often suboccipital and post-auricular, with a macular rash on the face, spreading to the trunk and proximal portions of the limbs; or serological evidence of rubella infection
consider: fever A03; other viral exanthem A76; generalized rash S07

A75 Infectious mononucleosis   *B27*

incl: glandular fever, M. Pfeiffer
criteria: inflammation of the tonsils/pharynx with lymphadenopathy not confined to the anterior cervical nodes, and either atypical lymphocytes on blood smear or splenomegaly; or abnormal heterophile antibody titre or Epstein–Barr virus titre
consider: fever A03; enlarged lymph nodes B02; acute upper respiratory tract infection R74

A76 Viral exanthem, other

A88.0, B03, B04, B08.0, B08.2 to B08.4, B08.8, B09

incl: cowpox, hand foot and mouth disease, fever with rash, fifth disease, roseola infantum

excl: measles A71; chickenpox A72; rubella A74; infectious mononucleosis A75

A77 Viral disease, other/NOS

A82, A90 to A96, A98, A99, B00.7, B25, B33.0, B33.1, B33.3, B33.8, B34, B97

incl: adenovirus, Coxsackie diseases, dengue fever, Ross River fever

excl: other viral exanthem A76; influenza R80

A78 Infectious disease, other/NOS

A20 to A28, A30, A31, A32, A38, A39.1 to A39.9, A40 to A44, A48.0, A48.2 to A48.4, A48.8, A49, A59.8, A59.9, A64, A68, A69.2, A69.8, A69.9, A70, A74.8, A74.9, A75, A77 to A79, B37.7 to B37.9, B38 to B43, B45 to B49, B55 to B57, B58.8, B58.9, B59, B60, B64, B89, B92, B94.8, B94.9, B95, B96, B99

incl: brucellosis, infection unspecified site, Lyme disease, mycoplasma, Q fever, rickettsial disease, scarlet fever, sexually transmitted disease NOS, thrush NOS, toxoplasmosis

excl: meningococcal meningitis N71

A79 Malignancy NOS

C38.1 to C38.3, C38.8, C45.7, C45.9, C46.7 to C46.9, C76, C78 to C80, C97, D09.7, D09.9

incl: secondary/metastatic neoplasm where primary site is unknown, carcinomatosis (unknown primary)

criteria: histological evidence of malignancy

consider: disease/condition of unspecified nature/site A99

A80 Trauma/injury NOS

S11, S15, S21, S25, S26, S27, S35, S37.9, S38.1, S38.3, S39.0, S39.8, S39.9, S45, S55, S65, S75, S85, S95, T11.4, T13.4, T14.5, T14.7 to T14.9, T28.4, T28.9

incl: road traffic accident

excl: multiple trauma A81; late effect of trauma A82

A81 Multiple trauma/injuries

S17.8, S17.9, S18, S19, S28, S29, S31.7, S36.7, S37.7, S37.8, S39, T00 to T05, T06.5, T06.8, T07, T29

incl: multiple internal injuries NOS

Note: In this classification 'general' or 'multiple' refers to three or more body sites or systems. Conditions affecting one or two sites should be coded to these sites.

A82 Secondary effect of trauma
T79.0 to T79.2, T79.4, T79.5, T79.7 to T79.9, T90 to T98

incl: deformity/scarring resulting from previous injury, old amputation
excl: effects related to specific body systems: code to system chapter; psychological effects of trauma/acute stress reaction P02; post-traumatic stress disorder P82; wound infection S11; scar of skin S99

A84 Poisoning by medical agent
T36 to T50

incl: toxic effect of overdose medical agent
excl: medication abuse P18; suicide attempt P77; insulin coma T87
criteria: toxicity/impairment produced by accidental/deliberate overdose of an agent that has remedial properties in its usual dosage

A85 Adverse effect medical agent
D61.1, D64.2, G44.4, I95.2, L27.0, L27.1, T88.6, T88.7

incl: side effects/allergy/anaphylaxis due to medication in proper dose
excl: poisoning by medical agent A84; reaction to immunization/transfusion A87; parkinsonism N87; medication abuse P18; contact dermatitis S88; insulin coma T87; analgesic nephropathy U88
criteria: symptom/complaint attributed to the proper use of medication, rather than due to disease or injury
Note: May also code the nature of the adverse effect.

A86 Toxic effect non-medicinal substance
D61.2, D64.2, T51 to T65

incl: general/local toxic effect carbon monoxide, industrial materials, lead, poisonous animals/insects/plants/snakes
excl: poisoning/adverse effect medical agent A84, A85; chronic/acute alcohol abuse P15, P16; tobacco abuse P17; medication abuse P18; drug abuse P19; respiratory toxic effects R99; non-toxic bites S12, S13; external chemical burns S14; contact dermatitis S88

A87 Complication of medical treatment
E89, G97, H59, H95, I97, J95, K91.0, K91.3, M96, N99, O29, O74, O86.0, O89, O90.0 to O90.2, T80, T81, T86, T87, T88.0 to T88.5, T88.8, T88.9

incl: anaesthetic shock, immunization/transfusion reaction, postoperative infection/haemorrhage/wound disruption, problems due to radiation for diagnosis/treatment
excl: poisoning by medical agent A84; adverse effects of medication A85; other hernia abdominalis D91; hypoglycaemia T87
criteria: an unexpected disorder resulting from surgical/medical/X-ray treatment/other medical management

A88 Adverse effect of physical factor
T33 to T35, T66 to T69, T70.2 to T70.4, T70.8, T70.9, T71, T73, T75, T78.8, T78.9

incl: adverse effect cold/heat/lightning/motion/pressure/radiation, chilblains, drowning, jetlag
excl: effect of medical radiation A87; snow blindness F79; effect of alcohol P15, P16; effect of tobacco P17; burn due to radiation S14; sunburn S80

A89 Effect of prosthetic device
K91.4, T82 to T85, Z43 to Z45, Z46.1 to Z46.9, Z93 to Z97

incl: discomfort/handicap/pain/limitation of function resulting from the fitting/ wearing of a device for supplying/amending deficiencies: catheter, colostomy, gastrostomy, heart valve, joint replacement, organ transplant, pacemaker
excl: effect denture/false teeth D19

A90 Congenital anomaly NOS/multiple
Q85 to Q87, Q89.3, Q89.4, Q89.7, Q89.9, Q90 to Q93, Q95 to Q99

incl: Down's syndrome, Marfan's syndrome, other chromosome abnormality, neurofibromatosis
excl: anomaly related to a specific body system to be coded to system chapter; congenital rubella A74

A91 Abnormal result investigation NOS
R73, R74, R76 to R79, R83 to R94

incl: abnormal unexplained pathology/imaging test, electrolyte disorder, hyperglycaemia
excl: unexplained abnormal white cells B84; other haematological abnormality B99; vitamin/nutritional deficiency T91; abnormal urine test U98; abnormal cervix smear X86
criteria: abnormal result not attributed to known disease

A92 Allergy/allergic reaction NOS   *T78.0 to T78.4*

incl: allergic oedema, anaphylactic shock, angioneurotic oedema, food allergy
excl: allergy resulting from medication A85; allergic rhinitis R97; urticaria S98

A93 Premature newborn   *P07*

criteria: live birth under 37 weeks' gestation

A94 Perinatal morbidity, other
P00 to P05, P08, P10 to P15, P20 to P29, P35 to P39, P50 to P61, P70 to P72, P74 to P78, P80, P81, P83, P90 to P94, P96

excl: congenital condition NOS A90; premature newborn A93; failure to thrive T10
criteria: morbidity originating in utero or within 7 days of birth

A95 Perinatal mortality *P95, R95*

criteria: death in utero or within 7 days of birth

A96 Death *R95, R96, R98, R99*

excl: perinatal death A95

A97 No disease *Z00, Z02*

incl: no illness/disease dealt with at encounter
excl: health maintenance/preventive medicine A98
Note: Sometimes a patient has a reason for encounter that the family doctor cannot interpret as a diagnosis within the domain of family practice. In these cases the FP/GP will use the code A97, indicating that the patient's reason for encounter refers to something the FP/GP cannot professionally respond to, except by explaining that this is the case.

A98 Health maintenance/preventive medicine
Z01, Z10 to Z13, Z23 to Z27, Z29, Z31.5, Z40, Z70

incl: medical procedure/counselling with a preventive purpose, including genetic counselling
excl: no disease A97

A99 Disease/condition of unspecified nature/site
D15.7, D15.9, D36.7, D36.9, D48.9, R69, Z03, Z04, Z08, Z09, Z22,
Z41, Z42, Z47 to Z54, Z71.0, Z71.2 to Z71.9, Z76.0 to Z76.4,
Z76.8, Z76.9, Z90.0, Z90.8, Z98.8

incl: disease carrier NOS, surveillance of ongoing problem NOS

B Blood, blood-forming organs, and immune mechanism

Component 1—Symptoms and complaints

B02 Lymph gland(s) enlarged/painful *R59*

incl: lymphadenopathy with/without pain/tenderness, other symptom/complaint lymph gland(s)
excl: acute lymphadenitis B70; chronic/non-specific lymphadenitis B71

B04 Blood symptom/complaint *R68.8*

excl: anaemia B82; pallor S08

B25 Fear of AIDS/HIV   *Z71.1*

excl: if the patient has the disease, code the disease
criteria: concern about/fear of AIDS/HIV in a patient without the disease/until the
            diagnosis is proven

B26 Fear of cancer blood/lymph   *Z71.1*

excl: if the patient has the disease, code the disease
criteria: concern about/fear of blood/lymph cancer in a patient without the
            disease/until the diagnosis is proven

B27 Fear of blood/lymph disease, other   *Z71.1*

excl: fear of cancer blood/lymph B26; if the patient has the disease, code the disease
criteria: concern about/fear of other blood/lymph disease in a patient without the
            disease/until the diagnosis is proven

B28 Limited function/disability (B)   *Z73.6*

incl: disability due to bleeding disorders
criteria: limitation of function/disability due to a problem of blood/blood-forming
            organs/immune mechanism
Note: The COOP/WONCA Charts are suitable for documenting the patient's functional
status (see Chapter 8).

B29 Lymph/immune mechanism symptom/complaint, other   *R68.8*

excl: splenomegaly B87

Component 7—Diagnoses/diseases

B70 Lymphadenitis, acute   *L04*

incl: abscess of lymph node
excl: chronic/non-specific/mesentric lymphadenitis B71; acute lymphangitis S76
criteria: one/more inflamed/enlarged and tender/painful lymph nodes in the same
            anatomical location, of recent onset (less than 6 weeks) and with unknown
            primary source of infection
consider: enlarged lymph node B02

B71 Lymphadenitis, chronic/non-specific   *I88*

incl: mesenteric lymphadenitis
excl: acute lymphadenitis B70; acute lymphangitis S76   *(cont.)*

criteria: enlarged tender lymph nodes present for more than 6 weeks; or demonstration of enlarged inflamed mesenteric lymph nodes by surgery/sonography/lymphography/otherwise
consider: enlarged lymph node B02

B72 Hodgkin's disease/lymphoma   C81 to C85

criteria: characteristic histological appearance
consider: other malignant neoplasm blood/lymph B74; benign/unspecified neoplasm blood/lymph B75

B73 Leukaemia   C91 to C95

incl: all types of leukaemia
criteria: characteristic histological appearance
consider: benign/unspecified neoplasm blood/lymph B75

B74 Malignant neoplasm blood, other   C37, C46.3, C77, C88, C90, C96

incl: myeloproliferative disease, multiple myeloma
excl: Hodgkin's disease/lymphoma B72

B75 Neoplasm blood, benign/unspecified   D15.0, D36.0, D45, D47

incl: benign neoplasm blood, neoplasm blood not specified as benign or malignant/when test is not available, polycythaemia rubra vera

B76 Ruptured spleen traumatic   S36.0

B77 Injury blood/lymph/spleen, other   T14.9

excl: ruptured spleen traumatic B76

B78 Hereditary haemolytic anaemia   D56 to D58

incl: sickle cell anaemia, sickle cell trait, spherocytosis, thalassaemia
criteria: characteristic findings by test such as haemoglobin electrophoresis, blood smear, or increased osmotic fragility of red cells
consider: other congenital anomaly blood/lymph B79

B79 Congenital anomaly blood/lymph, other
D61.0, D64.0, D64.4, Q89.0, Q89.8

incl: congenital anaemia
excl: hereditary haemolytic anaemia B78; haemophilia B83; haemangioma/lymphangioma S81

B80 Iron deficiency anaemia   *D50*

incl: anaemia due to blood loss
excl: iron deficiency without anaemia T91
criteria: decrease in haemoglobin or haematocrit below levels appropriate for age
             and sex; plus evidence of blood loss, or microcytic hypochromic red cells
             by appearance or indices in the absence of thalassaemia, or decreased
             serum iron and increased iron-binding capacity, or decreased serum
             ferritin, or reduced haemosiderin in bone marrow, or good response to iron
             administration
consider: other/unspecified anaemia B82

B81 Anaemia, vitamin B12/folate deficiency   *D51, D52*

incl: macrocytic anaemia, pernicious anaemia
excl: vit B12 deficiency without anaemia T91
criteria: macrocytic anaemia by smear/indices plus decreased vit B12/folate
             level/positive Schilling test

B82 Anaemia other/unspecified
D46, D53, D55, D59, D60, D61.3, D61.8, D61.9, D62, D63, D64.1,
D64.3, D64.8, D64.9

incl: acquired haemolytic anaemia, aplastic anaemia, blood autoimmune disease,
             megaloblastic anaemia NOS, protein deficiency anaemia
excl: iron deficiency anaemia B80; vit B12/folate deficiency anaemia B81;
             anaemia of pregnancy W84

B83 Purpura/coagulation defect   *D65 to D69*

incl: abnormal platelets, haemophilia, thrombocytopenia

B84 Unexplained abnormal white cells   *D70 to D72, R72*

incl: unexplained agranulocytosis, unexplained eosinophilia, unexplained leuko-
             cytosis, unexplained lymphocytosis, unexplained neutropenia
excl: leukaemia B73

B87 Splenomegaly   *R16.1, R16.2*

excl: hypersplenism B99

B90 HIV infection/AIDS   *B20 to B24, R75, Z21*

criteria: HIV infection proven in serological test in a patient with/without
             symptoms

B99 Blood/lymph/spleen disease, other
> *D73 to D77, D80 to D84, D86, D89, I89.1 to I89.9, R70, R71*

incl: complement defect, hypersplenism, immunodeficiency disorder, other/
          unspecified haematological abnormality, raised ESR, red cell abnormality,
          sarcoidosis, secondary polycythaemia
excl: lymphadenitis B70, B71; primary polycythemia B75; HIV/AIDS B90; lym-
          phoedema K99

D—Digestive

Component 1—Symptoms and complaints

D01 Abdominal pain/cramps, general   *R10.0, R10.4*

incl: abdominal colic, abdominal cramps/discomfort/pain NOS, infant colic
excl: epigastric ache D02; heartburn D03; other localized abdominal pain D06;
          dyspepsia/indigestion D07; flatulence/gas/belching D08; biliary colic D98;
          renal colic U14; dysmenorrhoea X02

D02 Abdominal pain, epigastric   *R10.1*

incl: epigastric discomfort, fullness, stomach ache/pain
excl: dyspepsia/indigestion D07; flatulence/gas/belching D08

D03 Heartburn   *R12*

incl: acidity, waterbrash
excl: epigastric pain D02; dyspepsia/indigestion D07; oesophagitis/reflux D84

D04 Rectal/anal pain   *K59.4, K62.8, R10.2, R10.3*

incl: anal spasm, proctalgia fugax
excl: impacted faeces D12

D05 Perianal itching   *L29.0, L29.3*

incl: perianal pruritus
excl: pruritus vulvae X16

D06 Abdominal pain, localized, other   *R10.1 to R10.3*

incl: colonic pain
excl: generalized abdominal pain D01; epigastric pain D02; heartburn D03; dyspepsia/
          indigestion D07; flatulence/gas/belching D08; irritable bowel syndrome
          D93; biliary colic D98; renal colic U14; dysmenorrhoea X02

D07 Dyspepsia/indigestion   *K30*

excl: epigastric pain D02; heartburn D03; flatulence/gas/belching D08

D08 Flatulence/gas/belching   *R14*

incl: bloating, eructation, gas pains, gaseous distension, passing wind
excl: dyspepsia/indigestion D07; change in abdominal size D25

D09 Nausea   *R11*

excl: feelings of over-eating D02; vomiting D10; alcohol-induced nausea P16;
             loss of appetite T03; nausea in pregnancy W05
Note: Code for nausea and vomiting as a diagnosis: D10

D10 Vomiting   *F50.5, R11*

incl: emesis, hyperemesis, retching
excl: haematemesis D14; vomiting in pregnancy W05
Note: Code for diarrhoea and vomiting as a diagnosis: D11

D11 Diarrhoea   *K52.9, K59.1*

incl: frequent/loose bowel movements, watery stools
excl: melaena D15; change in faeces/bowel movements D18

D12 Constipation   *K56.4, K59.0*

incl: faecal impaction
excl: ileus D99

D13 Jaundice   *R17*

incl: icterus

D14 Haematemesis/vomiting blood   *K92.0*

excl: haemoptysis R24

D15 Melaena   *K92.1*

incl: black/tarry stools
excl: fresh blood in stool D16

D16 Rectal bleeding   *K62.5*

incl: fresh blood in stool
excl: melaena D15

D17 Incontinence of bowel   *R15*

incl: faecal incontinence
excl: encopresis P13

D18 Change in faeces/bowel movements   *R19.4, R19.5*

excl: diarrhoea D11; constipation D12; incontinence of bowel D17

D19 Teeth/gum symptom/complaint   *K00.7, K08.8*

incl: denture problem, gingival inflammation/bleeding, teething, toothache
excl: caries D82

D20 Mouth/tongue/lip symptom/complaint
K13.1, K13.7, K14.5 to K14.9, R19.6, R68.2

incl: bad breath, coated tongue, cracked lips, dribbling, dry mouth, halitosis, sore
           mouth, swollen lips
excl: dental/gum problem D19; cheilosis D83; disturbance of taste N16; dehydra-
           tion T11

D21 Swallowing problem   *R13*

incl: choking feeling, dysphagia

D23 Hepatomegaly   *R16.0, R16.2*

D24 Abdominal mass NOS   *R19.0*

incl: lump abdomen
excl: splenomegaly B87; hepatomegaly D23; renal mass U14

D25 Abdominal distension   *R19.0*

incl: abdominal swelling without mass
excl: flatulence/gas/belching D08; abdominal mass D24; ascites D29

D26 Fear of cancer of digestive system   *Z71.1*

excl: if the patient has the disease, code the disease
criteria: concern about/fear of cancer of digestive system in a patient without the
              disease/until the diagnosis is proven

D27 Fear of digestive disease, other   *Z71.1*

excl: fear of cancer of digestive system D26; if the patient has the disease, code
           the disease   *(cont.)*

criteria: concern about/fear of other digestive disease in a patient without the
              disease/until the diagnosis is proven

D28 Limited function/disability (D)   *Z73.6*

excl: colostomy/gastrostomy A89; post-surgery disorder D99; dumping
              syndrome D99
criteria: limitation of function/disability due to a digestive problem
Note: The COOP/WONCA Charts are suitable for documenting the patient's functional
status (see Chapter 8).

D29 Digestive symptom/complaint, other
                                               K03.8, R11, R18, R19.1 to R19.3, R19.8

incl: ascites, teeth grinding

Component 7—Diagnosis/diseases

D70 Gastrointestinal infection   *A00 to A08*

incl: gastrointestinal infection/dysentery with specified organisms including
              campylobacter, giardia, salmonella, shigella, typhoid, cholera
excl: contact with/carrier of infective/parasitic disease A99; gastroenteritis pre-
              sumed infection D73
criteria: a symptomatic patient with isolation or serological evidence of patho-
              genic bacterium, virus, or protozoan from either the stool or from food
              ingested
consider: gastroenteritis presumed infection D73

D71 Mumps   *B26*

incl: mumps meningitis/orchitis/pancreatitis
criteria: acute non-suppurative, non-erythematous, diffuse tender inflammation of
              one or more salivary glands; or acute mumps infection demonstrated by culture
              or serology; or orchitis in a person exposed to mumps following appropriate
              incubation period
consider: swelling A08

D72 Viral hepatitis   *B15 to B19*

incl: all hepatitis presumed viral, chronic active hepatitis
excl: hepatitis NOS D97
criteria: evidence of viral infection with inflammation of the liver with/without jaun-
              dice; or serological evidence of an infection with a hepatitis virus
consider: jaundice D13; hepatomegaly D23

D73 Gastroenteritis, presumed infection   *A09*

incl: diarrhoea/vomiting presumed to be infective, dysentery NOS, food poisoning, gastric flu
excl: irritable bowel syndrome D93; non-infective enteritis and gastroenteritis D94, D99

D74 Malignant neoplasm stomach   *C16*

incl: carcinoma stomach
criteria: characteristic histological appearance
consider: other malignant digestive neoplasm (when primary site is unknown) D77; benign/unspecified digestive neoplasm D78

D75 Malignant neoplasm colon/rectum   *C18 to C21*

criteria: characteristic histological appearance
consider: other digestive malignant neoplasm (when primary site is unknown) D77; benign/unspecified digestive neoplasm D78

D76 Malignant neoplasm pancreas   *C25*

incl: carcinoma pancreas
criteria: characteristic histological appearance
consider: other malignant digestive neoplasm (when primary site is unknown) D77; benign/unspecified digestive neoplasm D78

D77 Malignant digestive neoplasm, other/NOS
C00 to C08, C14.8, C15, C17, C22 to C24, C26, C45.1, C46.2, C48

incl: all other primary malignancies of digestive system, gallbladder cancer, liver cancer
excl: malignancy of stomach, colon/rectum, pancreas D74–D76; secondary malignancy of known site (code to site); secondary malignancy of unknown site A79
consider: benign/unspecified digestive neoplasm D78

D78 Neoplasm digestive system, benign/unspecified
D00, D01, D10 to D13, D20, D37, D48.3, D48.4, K31.7, K62.0, K62.1

incl: benign digestive neoplasm, digestive neoplasm not specified as benign or malignant/when histology is not available, polyp of stomach, duodenum, colon, rectum

D79 Foreign body digestive system   *T18*

incl: foreign body swallowed/in digestive tract, including mouth, oesophagus, rectum
excl: foreign body in throat/inhaled R87

D80 Injury digestive system, other

S00.5, S01.5, S02.5, S03.2, S09.9, S10.0, S36.1 to S36.6, S36.8, S36.9, T28.0 to T28.2, T28.5 to T28.7

incl: injury to abdominal organ, teeth, tongue
excl: multiple organ injuries A81; injury pelvic organs X82, Y80

D81 Congenital anomaly digestive system   *Q18, Q35 to Q45*

incl: biliary anomaly, cleft lip/palate, Meckel's diverticulum, megacolon, Hirschsprung's disease, oesophageal atresia, pyloric stenosis, tongue-tie
excl: haemangioma/lymphangioma S81; congenital metabolic disorder T80

D82 Teeth/gum disease   *K00.0 to K00.6, K00.8, K00.9, K01 to K10*

incl: caries, dental abscess, gingivitis, malocclusion, temporomandibular joint disorder
excl: teething/denture problem D19; injury to teeth/gum D80; Vincent's angina D83

D83 Mouth/tongue/lip disease

A69.0, A69.1, B37.0, K11, K12, K13.0, K13.2 to K13.7, K14.0 to K14.4, K14.8, K14.9

incl: aphthous ulcer, cheilosis, glossitis, mucocoele, oral thrush, parotitis, salivary calculus, stomatitis, Vincent's angina
excl: mumps D71; other injury digestive system D80; herpes simplex S71

D84 Oesophagus disease   *K20 to K23*

incl: achalasia, oesophagial diverticulum, Mallory–Weiss syndrome, oesophagitis, oesophagus ulceration, reflux
excl: cancer of oesophagus D77; hiatus hernia D90; oesophageal varices K99

D85 Duodenal ulcer   *K26*

incl: bleeding/obstructing/perforated ulcer
criteria: characteristic imaging findings; or characteristic endoscopy findings; or exacerbation of symptoms in a patient with a previously proven duodenal ulcer
consider: heartburn D03; dyspepsia/indigestion D07

D86 Peptic ulcer, other   *E16.4, K25, K27, K28*

incl: gastric/gastrojejunal/marginal ulcer, acute erosion, Zollinger–Ellison syndrome
excl: oesophageal ulcer D84; duodenal ulcer D85
criteria: characteristic imaging/endoscopy findings; or exacerbation of symptoms in a patient with a previously proven ulcer
consider: heartburn D03; dyspepsia/indigestion D07

D87 Stomach function disorder   *K29, K31.0 to K31.6, K31.8, K31.9*

incl: acute dilatation stomach, duodenitis, gastritis
excl: gastrointestinal infection D70; gastroenteritis presumed infection D73
criteria: disorder of stomach function proven by investigation
consider: abdominal pain D01, D06; epigastric pain D02; heartburn D03; indigestion/
dyspepsia D07; gas problems (wind) D08; nausea D09; vomiting D10;
oesophagitis D84

D88 Appendicitis   *K35 to K37*

incl: appendix abscess/perforation
criteria: objective evidence of inflammation of the appendix, such as demonstrated at
operation or pathological examination
consider: abdominal pain D01, D06; vomiting D10

D89 Inguinal hernia   *K40*

excl: femoral hernia D91
criteria: swelling in the inguinal region and transmitted impulse with cough, or
enlargement on straining, or swelling reducible into the abdomen, or intestinal obstruction
consider: abdominal mass D24

D90 Hiatus hernia   *K44*

incl: diaphragmatic hernia
excl: oesophagitis/reflux D84
criteria: characteristic findings on imaging/endoscopy/intraluminal pressure studies/
surgery
consider: epigastric pain D02; heartburn D03; dyspepsia/indigestion D07

D91 Abdominal hernia, other   *K41 to K43, K45, K46*

incl: femoral/umbilical/ventral hernia
excl: post-surgical hernia A87; hiatus inguinalis D89; hiatus hernia D90
criteria: demonstration at surgery; or swelling in the specified area and transmitted
impulse with cough, or enlargement on straining, or reducible into the
abdomen, or intestinal obstruction
consider: abdominal mass D24

D92 Diverticular disease   *K57*

incl: diverticulitis/diverticulosis of intestine
excl: Meckel's diverticulum D81; oesophageal diverticulum D84
criteria: imaging demonstration of diverticula; or demonstration of diverticula at surgery;
or acute abdominal pain with fever and palpable tender descending/sigmoid colon
consider: abdominal pain D01, D06

D93 Irritable bowel syndrome   *K58*

incl: mucous colitis, spastic colon
excl: gastrointestinal infection D70; gastroenteritis presumed infection D73;
            regional enteritis D94; vascular insufficiency of gut, allergic/dietetic/toxic
            gastroenteritis/colitis D99; psychogenic diarrhoea P75
criteria: continuous/intermittent abdominal pain and variable bowel pattern over a
            period of time; and increased gas, or tender and palpable colon, or history of
            mucous without blood in stool
consider: abdominal pain D01, D06; flatulence D08; diarrhoea D11; constipation D12

D94 Chronic enteritis/ulcerative colitis   *K50, K51, K52.0*

incl: Crohn's disease, regional enteritis, ulcerative colitis
criteria: characteristic endoscopic/imaging/histological findings
consider: abdominal pain D01, D06; diarrhoea D11; mucous colitis D93

D95 Anal fissure/perianal abscess   *K60, K61*

incl: anal fistula, ischiorectal abscess
excl: pilonidal abscess S85

D96 Worms/other parasites   *B65 to B83*

incl: cestodes, creeping eruption, intestinal parasites unspecified, trichiniasis,
            hydatid disease
criteria: either demonstration of helminth in adult form, larvae, or ova; or positive
            skin tests; or positive serology

D97 Liver disease NOS   *B58.1, B94.2, K70 to K77*

incl: alcohol hepatitis, cirrhosis, fatty liver, hepatitis NOS, liver failure, portal
            hypertension
excl: viral hepatitis D72; hydatid disease D96

D98 Cholecystitis/cholelithiasis   *K80 to K83, K87.0*

incl: biliary colic, cholangitis, gallstones
criteria: *cholecystitis*: demonstration of typical pathology by ultrasonography or
            surgery; or localized right upper quadrant tenderness and jaundice or fever
            or history of gallstones;
            cholelithiasis: imaging or surgical demonstration of gallstones;
            acute biliary colic: acute colicky right upper quadrant abdominal pain
            without fever; and jaundice or right upper quadrant abdominal tenderness, or
            history of gallstones
consider: localized abdominal pain D06

D99 Disease digestive system, other
> *K38, K52.1, K52.2, K52.8, K52.9, K55, K56.0 to K56.3, K56.5 to K56.7, K59.2, K59.3, K59.8, K59.9, K62.2 to K62.4, K62.6 to K62.9, K63, K65 to K67, K85, K86, K87.1, K90, K91.1, K91.2, K91.5 to K91.9, K92.2, K92.8, K92.9, K93, Z90.3, Z90.4, Z98.0*

incl: abdominal adhesions, coeliac disease, dumping syndrome, food intolerance, allergic/toxic/dietetic gastroenteropathy, ileus, intestinal obstruction, intussusception, lactose intolerance, malabsorption syndrome, mesenteric vascular disease, pancreatic disease, peritonitis, secondary megacolon, sprue

excl: antibiotic-associated colitis A85; malignancy digestive system D74–D77

F Eye

Component 1—Symptoms and complaints

F01 Eye pain   *H57.1*

excl: abnormal eye sensations F13

F02 Red eye   *H57.8*

incl: bloodshot/inflamed eye

F03 Eye discharge   *H04.2*

incl: lacrimation, purulent discharge, watery eye

F04 Visual floaters/spots   *H53.1*

incl: fixed/floating spots in the visual field
excl: other visual disturbance F05

F05 Visual disturbance, other   *H53.1 to H53.3, H53.8, H53.9, H54.7*

incl: blurred vision, difficulty reading, diplopia, eye strain, photophobia, scotoma and dazzle when symptoms confined to eyes, temporary blindness NOS, visual loss, weak eyes
excl: blindness one eye F28; snow blindness F79; refractive errors F91; permanent blindness F94; colour/night blindness F99

F13 Eye sensation abnormal   *H57.8*

incl: burning/dry/itchy eye
excl: eye pain F01

F14 Eye movements abnormal   *H55*

incl: abnormal blinking, lazy eye, nystagmus
excl: squint F95; twitching N08; tic of eye P10

F15 Eye appearance abnormal   *H57.8*

incl: change eye colour, swollen eye
excl: red eye F02

F16 Eyelid symptom/complaint   *H02.2 to H02.9*

incl: ptosis eyelid
excl: inflamed eyelid F72

F17 Glasses symptom/complaint   *Z46.0*

incl: problems due to spectacles affecting structure, function, or sensations of
           eye(s)
excl: contact lens symptom/complaint F18

F18 Contact lens symptom/complaint   *Z46.0*

incl: problems due to contact lens affecting structure, function, or sensations of
           eye(s)

F27 Fear of eye disease   *Z71.1*

incl: fear of blindness
excl: if the patient has the disease, code the disease
criteria: concern about/fear of eye disease in a patient without the disease/until the
           diagnosis is proven

F28 Limited function/disability (F)   *H54.4 to H54.6, Z73.6*

incl: blindness one eye
excl: blindness F94
criteria: limitation of function/disability due to a problem with vision/eye(s)
Note: The COOP/WONCA Charts are suitable for documenting the patient's functional
status (see Chapter 8).

F29 Eye symptom/complaint, other   *H57.9*

Component 7—Diagnosis/diseases

F70 Conjunctivitis, infectious
                          A74.0, B30, H10.0, H10.2 to H10.5, H10.8, H10.9, H13

incl: bacterial/viral conjunctivitis, conjunctivitis NOS   *(cont.)*

excl: allergic conjunctivitis with/without rhinorrhoea F71; flash burn F79; trachoma F86
criteria: presumed or proven infectious inflammation of conjunctiva

F71 Conjunctivitis, allergic   *H10.1*

incl: allergic conjunctivitis with/without rhinorrhoea
excl: bacterial/viral conjunctivitis F70; flashburn F79; trachoma F86
criteria: presumed or proven hyperaemia of conjunctiva, excess watering of eyes, itching/oedema of conjunctiva

F72 Blepharitis/stye/chalazion   *H00, H01*

incl: dermatitis/dermatosis of eyelids, eyelid infection, hordeolum, meibomian cyst, tarsal cyst
excl: dacryocystitis F73
criteria: generalized/localized inflammation/swelling of eyelid/tarsal gland

F73 Eye infection/inflammation, other
B00.5, B58.0, H03, H04.3, H04.4, H05.0, H05.1, H16.1 to H16.4, H16.8, H16.9, H20 to H22, H30, H32

incl: dacryocystitis, herpes simplex of eye without corneal ulcer, inflammation of the orbit, iritis, iridocyclitis, keratitis
excl: measles keratitis A71; corneal ulcer (herpes) F85; trachoma F86; herpes zoster S70

F74 Neoplasm of eye/adnexa   *C69, D09.2, D31, D48.7*

incl: benign/malignant neoplasm of eye/adnexa

F75 Contusion/haemorrhage, eye   *H11.3, H57.8, S00.1, S05.1*

incl: black eye, hyphaema, subconjunctival haemorrhage
excl: corneal ulcer F85

F76 Foreign body in eye   *T15*

excl: corneal abrasion F79

F79 Injury eye, other   *H16.1, H44.6, H44.7, S00.2, S01.1, S05.0, S05.2 to S05.9, S09.9, T26*

incl: corneal abrasion, flash burn, snow blindness
excl: contusion/haemorrhage eye F75; foreign body in eye F76

F80 Blocked lacrimal duct of infant   *Q10.5*

excl: dacryocystitis F73; blocked lacrimal duct in older person F99
criteria: overflow of tears without crying, beginning before the age of 3 months

F81 Congenital anomaly eye, other   *Q10.0 to Q10.4, Q10.6, Q10.7, Q11 to Q15*

F82 Detached retina   *H33*

F83 Retinopathy   *H35.0 to H35.2, H35.4, H36*

incl: diabetic/hypertensive retinopathy
Note: Double code known causative disease, e.g. diabetes T89, T90 or hypertension K87.

F84 Macular degeneration   *H35.3*

excl: retinopathy F83

F85 Corneal ulcer   *H16.0, H19*

incl: dendritic ulcer, viral keratitis
excl: corneal abrasion/other eye injury F79

F86 Trachoma   *A71, B94.0*

criteria: either proven infection with *Chlamydia trachomatis*, or typical clinical fea-
            tures including chronic inflammation and hypertrophy of the conjunctiva
            with formation of yellowish/greyish granules
consider: red eye F02; discharge from eye F03

F91 Refractive error   *H52*

incl: astigmatism, hypermetropia, long-sightedness, myopia, presbyopia, short-
            sightedness
excl: partial/complete blindness F94
criteria: visual deficit correctible with an appropriate lens

F92 Cataract   *H25, H26, H28*

excl: congenital cataract F81
criteria: opacity of part/all of the optic lens that reduces/impairs vision

F93 Glaucoma   *H40, H42*

incl: raised intraocular pressure
excl: congenital glaucoma F81

F94 Blindness   *H54.0 to H54.3*

incl: partial/complete blindness of both eyes
excl: blurred vision/temporary blindness F05; blindness one eye F28; snow blind-
            ness F79; refractive errors F91; colour/night blindness F99

F95 Strabismus   *H49 to H51*

incl: cross-eye, squint
criteria: lack of parallelism of visual axis of the eyes demonstrated at medical
           examination
consider: abnormal eye movement F14

F99 Eye/adnexa disease, other
           H02.0, H02.1, H02.8, H02.9, H04.0, H04.1, H04.5 to H04.9, H05.2 to H05.5,
           H05.8, H05.9, H06, H11.0 to H11.2, H11.4, H11.8, H11.9, H15, H17,
           H18, H27, H31, H34, H35.5 to H35.9, H43, H44.0 to H44.5,
           H44.8, H44.9, H45 to H48, H53.0, H53.4 to H53.6, H53.8,
           H57.0, H57.8, H58

incl: amblyopia, arcus senilis, colour blindness, corneal opacity, disorder of orbit,
           ectropion, entropion, episcleritis, ingrowing eyelash, night blindness, papil-
           loedema, pterygium, scleritis

H Ear

Component 1—Symptoms and complaints

H01 Ear pain/earache   *H92.0*

H02 Hearing complaint   *H93.2*

excl: deafness one ear H86; deafness both ears H86

H03 Tinnitus, ringing/buzzing ear   *H93.1*

incl: echo in ear
excl: ears crackling/popping H29

H04 Ear discharge   *H92.1*

excl: blood in/from ear H05

H05 Bleeding ear   *H92.2*

incl: blood in/from ear

H13 Plugged feeling ear   *H93.8*

incl: blocked ear
excl: excessive ear wax H81

H15 Concern with appearance of ears
R46.8

excl: bat ears/congenital anomaly ear H80

H27 Fear of ear disease
Z71.1

incl: fear of deafness
excl: in a patient with the disease, code the disease
criteria: concern about/fear of ear disease/deafness in a patient without the disease/until the diagnosis is proven

H28 Limited function/disability (H)
Z73.6

incl: temporary deafness
excl: presbyacusis H84; acoustic trauma H85; deafness H86; dizziness/vertigo N17
criteria: limitation of function/disability due to a problem with ear/hearing
Note: The COOP/WONCA Charts are suitable for documenting the patient's functional status (see Chapter 8).

H29 Ear symptom/complaint, other
H93.9

incl: ears crackling/popping, itchy ears, pulling at ears
excl: dizziness/loss of balance/vertigo N17

Component 7—Diagnosis/diseases

H70 Otitis externa
H60, H62

incl: abscess/eczema/furuncle external auditory meatus, swimmer's ear
criteria: inflammation/desquamation of the external auditory canal

H71 Acute otitis media/myringitis

H66.0, H66.4, H66.9, H67, H70.0, H73.0

incl: acute suppurative otitis media, otitis media NOS, acute mastoiditis, acute tympanitis
excl: serous otitis media H72; chronic otitis media H74
criteria: recent perforation of the tympanic membrane discharging pus; or inflamed and bulging tympanic membrane; or one ear drum more red than the other; or red tympanic membrane, with ear pain; or bullae on the tympanic membrane
consider: ear pain H01; ear discharge H04

H72 Serous otitis media
H65

incl: glue ear, otitis media with effusion (OME)
(cont.)

excl: acute otitis media H71; chronic otitis media H74
criteria: visible fluid behind the tympanic membrane, without inflammation; or dullness of the tympanic membrane with either retracting, bulging, or with related impairment of hearing
consider: plugged feeling ear H13; eustachian salpingitis/block H73

H73 Eustachian salpingitis *H68, H69*

incl: eustachian block/catarrh/dysfunction
excl: serous otitis media H72
consider: plugged feeling ear H13

H74 Chronic otitis media *H66.1 to H66.3, H70.1 to H70.9, H71, H73.1, H75*

incl: cholesteatoma, chronic suppurative otitis media, chronic mastoiditis
excl: serous otitis media H72

H75 Neoplasm of ear *C30.1, D14.0, D38.5, D48.1, D48.5*

incl: benign/malignant neoplasm of ear
excl: polyp ear H99; acoustic neuroma N75

H76 Foreign body in ear *T16*

H77 Perforation, ear drum *H72*

excl: perforation ear drum with infection H71, H74; traumatic/pressure rupture ear drum H79

H78 Superficial injury of ear *S00.4*

incl: external meatus/pinna injury
excl: injury of tympanic membrane H79

H79 Ear injury, other *S01.3, S07.0, S08.1, S09.2, S09.8, S09.9, T70.0*

incl: traumatic/pressure rupture of ear drum

H80 Congenital anomaly of ear *Q16, Q17*

incl: accessory auricle, bat ears
excl: congenital deafness H86

H81 Excessive ear wax *H61.2*

criteria: symptom/complaint due to wax in ear canal

H82 Vertiginous syndrome   *A88.1, H81, H82, H83.0*

incl: benign paroxysmal/positional vertigo, labyrinthitis, Ménière's disease,
            vestibular neuronitis
criteria: true rotational vertigo
consider: vertigo/giddiness/dizziness N17

H83 Otosclerosis   *H80*

H84 Presbyacusis   *H91.1*

excl: deafness H86
criteria: gradual onset with ageing of symmetrical, bilateral deafness, particularly
            involving high-frequency sounds
consider: hearing impairment H28

H85 Acoustic trauma   *H83.3*

incl: noise deafness
excl: perforation of ear drum H77
criteria: deafness in the high-frequency range with a definite history of exposure to
            loud noise
consider: hearing impairment H28; deafness H86

H86 Deafness   *H90, H91.0, H91.2 to H91.9*

incl: congenital deafness, deafness one ear, partial/complete deafness both ears
excl: temporary deafness H28; otosclerosis H83; presbyacusis H84; noise deaf-
            ness H85

H99 Ear/mastoid disease, other
                H61.0, H61.1, H61.3 to H61.9, H73.8, H73.9, H74, H83.1, H83.2, H83.8,
                            H83.9, H93.0, H93.3, H93.8, H94

incl: polyp of middle ear
excl: mastoiditis H74

K Circulatory

Component 1—Symptoms and complaints

K01 Heart pain   *R07.2*

incl: pain attributed to the heart
excl: chest pain NOS A11; fear of heart attack K24; angina pectoris K74; chest
            tightness R29

K02 Pressure/tightness of heart *R07.2*

incl: heaviness of heart
excl: chest pain NOS A11; fear of heart attack K24; angina pectoris K74; shortness
of breath/dyspnoea R02

K03 Cardiovascular pain NOS *R09.8*

excl: pain attributed to the heart K01; claudication K92; migraine N89

K04 Palpitations/awareness of heart *R00.0 to R00.2*

incl: tachycardia
excl: paroxysmal tachycardia K79

K05 Irregular heartbeat, other *R00.8*

excl: palpitations K04

K06 Prominent veins *I78.1, I87.8*

incl: unusually prominent veins, spider naevus
excl: varicose veins K95; haemangioma S81

K07 Swollen ankles/oedema *R60*

incl: dropsy, fluid retention, swollen feet/legs
excl: ankle symptom L16; localized swelling S04

K22 Risk factor for cardiovascular disease *Z82.3, Z82.4, Z86.7*

incl: personal/family history, previous episode, other risk factor for cardiovascular
disease

K24 Fear of heart disease *Z71.1*

incl: fear of heart attack
excl: if the patient has the disease, code the disease
criteria: concern about/fear of heart attack/disease in a patient without the disease/
until the diagnosis is proven

K25 Fear of hypertension *Z71.1*

excl: if the patient has the disease, code the disease
criteria: concern about/fear of hypertension in a patient without the disease/until the
diagnosis is proven

K27 Fear of cardiovascular disease, other   *Z71.1*

excl: fear of cardiovascular diseases K24, K25; if the patient has the disease, code
            the disease
criteria: concern about/fear of other disease of the circulatory system in a patient
            without the disease/until the diagnosis is proven

K28 Limited function/disability (K)   *Z73.6*

criteria: limitation of function/disability due to a cardiovascular problem
Note: The COOP/WONCA Charts are suitable for documenting the patient's functional
status (see Chapter 8).

K29 Cardiovascular symptom/complaint, other   *R03.1, R09.8*

incl: heart trouble, low blood pressure, weak heart
excl: fluid in chest R82; cyanosis S08

Component 7—Diagnosis/diseases

K70 Infection of circulatory system   *A39.5, B33.2, B37.6, I30, I32, I33, I38 to I41*

incl: acute/subacute endocarditis, bacterial endocarditis, myocarditis, pericarditis
            (other than rheumatic)
excl: rheumatic heart disease K71; phlebitis/thrombophlebitis K94; arteritis K99

K71 Rheumatic fever/heart disease   *I00 to I02, I05 to I09*

incl: chorea, mitral stenosis
criteria: *Acute rheumatic fever*: two major, or one major, and two minor manifesta-
            tions, plus evidence of preceding streptococcal infection;
            Major manifestations: migratory polyarthritis; carditis; chorea; erythema
            marginatum; subcutaneous nodules of recent onset;
            Minor manifestations: fever; arthralgia; raised ESR or positive C-reactive
            protein; prolonged P-R interval on ECG;
            Chronic rheumatic heart disease: either physical findings consistent with
            a valve lesion of the heart in a patient with a history of rheumatic fever;
            or physical findings consistent with mitral stenosis, even in the absence
            of a history of rheumatic fever, but without any other demonstrable
            cause
consider: heart valve disease K83; other heart disease K84

K72 Neoplasm cardiovascular   *C38.0, C45.2, D15.1, D15.2, D48.7*

incl: benign/malignant cardiovascular neoplasm
excl: haemangioma S81

K73 Congenital anomaly cardiovascular   *I42.4, Q20 to Q28*

incl: atrial/ventricular septal defect, Fallot's tetralogy, patent ductus arteriosus
excl: haemangioma S81

K74 Ischaemic heart disease with angina   *I20, I24.0, I24.8, I24.9*

incl: angina of effort, angina pectoris, angina with spasm, ischaemic chest pain,
            unstable angina
excl: ischaemic heart disease without angina K76
criteria: history plus ECG or imaging evidence of old myocardial infarction; or
            demonstration of myocardial ischaemia by resting or exercise ECG; or
            investigatory evidence of coronary artery narrowing or ventricular aneurysm
consider: heart pain K01

K75 Acute myocardial infarction   *I21 to I23, I24.1*

incl: myocardial infarction specified as acute or within 4 weeks (28 days) of onset
excl: old/healed myocardial infarction K74, K76
criteria: chest pain characteristic of myocardial ischaemia, lasting more than 15 min,
            and/or abnormal ST-T changes or new Q waves in electrocardiogram or
            raised blood cardiac enzymes
consider: heart pain K01; angina pectoris K74; chronic ischaemic heart disease K76
Note: Double code K74 or K76 as well.

K76 Ischaemic heart disease without angina   *I25*

incl: aneurysm of heart, arteriosclerotic/atherosclerotic heart disease, coronary
            artery disease, ischaemic cardiomyopathy, old myocardial infarction, silent
            myocardial ischaemia
excl: ischaemic heart disease with angina K74
criteria: history plus ECG, or imaging evidence of old myocardial infarction; or
            demonstration of myocardial ischaemia by resting or exercise ECG; or
            investigation evidence of coronary artery narrowing; or ventricular aneurysm

K77 Heart failure   *I50*

incl: cardiac asthma, congestive heart failure, heart failure NOS, left ventricular
            failure, pulmonary oedema, right ventricular failure
excl: cor pulmonale K82
criteria: multiple signs including dependent oedema, raised jugular venous pressure,
            hepatomegaly in the absence of liver disease, pulmonary congestion, pleural
            effusion, enlarged heart

K78 Atrial fibrillation/flutter   *I48*

excl: paroxysmal tachycardia K79   *(cont.)*

criteria: characteristic findings on electrocardiogram; or totally irregular heart rate
              with a pulse deficit
consider: palpitations K04; abnormal irregular heartbeat K05

K79 Paroxysmal tachycardia   *147*

incl: supraventricular/ventricular tachycardia
excl: tachycardia NOS K04; atrial fibrillation K78
criteria: history of recurrent episodes of rapid heart rate (over 140/min) with both
              abrupt onset and termination
consider: palpitations K04; abnormal irregular heartbeat K05

K80 Cardiac arrhythmia NOS   *149*

incl: atrial/junctional/ventricular premature beats, bradycardia, bigeminy, ectopic
              beats, extrasystoles, premature beats, sick sinus syndrome, ventricular
              fibrillation/flutter
excl: paroxysmal tachycardia K79
criteria: one or more heart beats that occur at times other than the regular beats of the
              underlying rhythm
consider: palpitations K04, abnormal irregular heartbeat K05

K81 Heart/arterial murmur NOS   *R01, R09.8*

incl: cardiac/carotid/renal artery bruit, innocent murmur of childhood
excl: rheumatic heart disease K71; valve disease K83; cerebrovascular disease K90

K82 Pulmonary heart disease   *I27, I28*

incl: chronic cor pulmonale, disease of pulmonary vessels, primary pulmonary
              hypertension
excl: pulmonary embolism K93
criteria: presence of a chronic disease of the lungs, pulmonary vasculature, or respira-
              tory gas exchange; plus presence of right ventricular enlargement or right
              heart failure
consider: right heart failure K77

K83 Heart valve disease NOS   *I34 to I37*

incl: chronic endocarditis, mitral valve prolapse, non-rheumatic aortic/mitral/pul-
              monary/tricuspid valve disorder
excl: rheumatic valve disease K71
criteria: absence of criteria for chronic rheumatic heart disease K71; plus evidence of
              valvular dysfunction by either characteristic heart murmur, or by
              imaging/echocardiographic evidence of abnormal valve
consider: hypertensive heart disease K87; cardiac murmur NOS K81

K84 Heart disease, other   *I31, I42.0 to I42.3, I42.5 to I42.9, I43 to I46, I51, I52, O90.3*

incl: bundle branch block, cardiac arrest, cardiomegaly, disease of pericardium, cardiomyopathy, heart block, left bundle-branch block, other conduction disorders
excl: cardiac arrhythmia K80

K85 Elevated blood pressure   *R03.0*

incl: elevated blood pressure not meeting criteria for K86 and K87, transient/labile hypertension

K86 Hypertension, uncomplicated   *I10*

incl: essential hypertension, hypertension NOS, idiopathic hypertension
excl: hypertension with complications K87; hypertension in pregnancy W81
criteria: either two or more readings per encounter, taken at two or more encounters, with blood pressures that average over 95 mmHg diastolic or over 160 mmHg systolic in adult patients; or two or more readings at a single encounter with an average diastolic blood pressure of 120 mmHg or more; plus absence of evidence of secondary involvement of heart, kidney, eye, or brain
consider: elevated blood pressure K85
Notes: (1) For children, consult appropriate paediatric blood pressure tables. (2) If secondary hypertension, code also the underlying cause.

K87 Hypertension, complicated   *I11 to I13, I15, I67.4*

incl: malignant hypertension
excl: uncomplicated hypertension K86
criteria: either two or more readings per encounter, taken at two or more encounters, with blood pressures that average over 95 mmHg diastolic or over 160 mmHg systolic in adult patients; or two or more readings at a single encounter with an average diastolic blood pressure of 120 mmHg or more; plus evidence of abnormalities of the heart (enlargement, failure), kidney (albuminuria, azotaemia), eye, or brain attributed to hypertension
Note: (1) For children, consult appropriate paediatric blood pressure tables. (2) If secondary hypertension, code also the underlying cause.

K88 Postural hypotension   *I95.0, I95.1, I95.8, I95.9*

incl: idiopathic/orthostatic hypotension
excl: hypotension due to drugs A85
criteria: signs or symptoms of cerebrovascular insufficiency (dizziness, syncope) on changing from the supine to the upright position; and a fall in mean blood pressure of 15 mmHg on two or more occasions when changing from the supine to the upright position
consider: low blood pressure K29

K89 Transient cerebral ischaemia   *G45*

incl: basilar insufficiency, drop attacks, transient ischaemic attack (TIA), transient
            global amnesia
excl: carotid bruit K81; cerebrovascular accident K90; migraine N89
criteria: symptoms of transient (less than 24 h) hypofunction of the brain, with sudden
            onset, presumed of vascular origin, without sequelae, and with exclusion of
            migraine/migraine equivalent/epilepsy
consider: fainting/syncope A06
Note: Double code with K91.

K90 Stroke/cerebrovascular accident   *G46, I60 to I64*

incl: apoplexy, cerebral embolism/infarction/thrombosis/occlusion/stenosis/
            haemorrhage, cerebrovascular accident (CVA), subarachnoid haemorrhage
excl: transient cerebral ischaemia K89; traumatic intracranial haemorrhage N80
criteria: signs and symptoms of a disturbance of cerebral function, presumed of
            vascular origin, lasting more than 24 h or causing death, and within 4 weeks
            (28 days) of onset
Note: Double code with K91.

K91 Cerebrovascular disease   *I65, I66, I67.0 to I67.3, I67.5 to I67.9, I68, I69*

incl: cerebral aneurysm, sequelae of stroke
criteria: previous transient cerebral ischaemia/stroke; or investigation evidence of
            cerebrovascular disease

K92 Atherosclerosis/peripheral vascular disease   *I70, I73, I74, R02*

incl: arteriosclerosis, arterial embolism/thrombosis/stenosis, atheroma, endarteritis,
            gangrene, intermittent claudication, limb ischaemia, Raynaud's syndrome,
            vasospasm
excl: mesenteric atherosclerosis D99; ophthalmic/retinal atherosclerosis F99;
            coronary atherosclerosis K74 to K76; pulmonary atherosclerosis K82; cere-
            bral atherosclerosis K89, K90; aneurysm K99; renal atherosclerosis U99

K93 Pulmonary embolism   *I26*

incl: pulmonary (artery/vein) infarction, thromboembolism, thrombosis
criteria: sudden onset of dyspnoea/tachypnoea and either clinical or imaging evidence
            of pulmonary infarction, or ECG evidence of acute right ventricular strain
consider: dyspnoea R02

K94 Phlebitis/thrombophlebitis   *I80 to I82, I87.0, I87.8*

incl: superficial/deep vein thrombosis, phlebothrombosis, portal thrombosis
excl: cerebral thrombosis K89, K90

K95 Varicose veins of leg
I83.1, I83.9, I87.2

incl: varicose eczema, venous insufficiency, venous stasis
excl: varicose ulcer S97
criteria: presence of dilated superficial veins in lower extremities; or demonstration of valve incompetence of veins
consider: prominent veins K06

K96 Haemorrhoids
I84

incl: internal haemorrhoids with/without complications, perianal haematoma, piles, residual haemorrhoidal skin tag, thrombosed external haemorrhoids, varicose veins of anus/rectum
criteria: visualization of varicosities of the venous plexus of the anus or canal; or tender, painful, blue-coloured localized swelling of acute onset, in the perianal area; or skin tags in the perianal area
consider: anal pain D04; rectal bleeding D16; anal lump D29

K99 Cardiovascular disease, other
I71, I72, I77, I78.0, I78.8, I78.9, I79, I85, I86, I87.1, I87.9, I89.0, I98, I99, M30, M31, R57, T06.3

incl: aortic aneurysm, arteriovenous fistula, arteritis, lymphoedema, oesophageal varices, other aneurysm, polyarteritis nodosa, vasculitis, varicose veins of sites other than lower extremities
excl: chronic/non-specific lymphadenitis B71; cerebral aneurysm K91; gangrene K92

L Musculoskeletal

Component 1—Symptoms and complaints

L01 Neck symptom/complaint
M54.0, M54.2

incl: pain attributed to cervical spine/musculoskeletal system
excl: headache N01; pain in face N03

L02 Back symptom/complaint
M54.0, M54.6, M54.8, M54.9

incl: backache NOS, thoracic back pain
excl: low back pain L03

L03 Low back symptom/complaint
M53.3, M54.0, M54.5

incl: back pain (lumbar/sacroiliac), coccydynia, lumbago, lumbalgia
excl: thoracic back pain L02; sciatica L86

L04 Chest symptom/complaint   *R07.3, R29.8*

incl: chest pain attributed to musculoskeletal system
excl: chest pain NOS A11; pain attributed to the heart K01; painful respiration/
           pleuritic pain/pleurodynia R01

L05 Flank/axilla symptom/complaint   *R29.8*

incl: loin pain
excl: kidney symptom U14

L07 Jaw symptom/complaint   *K07.6, R25.2, R29.8*

incl: temporomandibular joint symptom
excl: teeth/gum symptom/complaint D19

L08 Shoulder symptom/complaint   *M25.4 to M25.6*

L09 Arm symptom/complaint   *M79.6, R25.2, R29.8*

excl: muscle pain/myalgia L18

L10 Elbow symptom/complaint   *M25.4 to M25.6*

L11 Wrist symptom/complaint   *M25.4 to M25.6*

L12 Hand/finger symptom/complaint   *M25.4 to M25.6, M79.6, R25.2, R29.8*

L13 Hip symptom/complaint   *M25.4 to M25.6, R29.4*

L14 Leg/thigh symptom/complaint   *M79.6, R25.2, R29.8*

incl: leg cramps
excl: muscle pain/myalgia L18; restless legs N04

L15 Knee symptom/complaint   *M25.4 to M25.6*

L16 Ankle symptom/complaint   *M25.4 to M25.6*

L17 Foot/toe symptom/complaint
                           M25.4 to M25.6, M77.4, M77.5, M79.6, R25.2, R29.8

incl: metatarsalgia

L18 Muscle pain   *M60.1, M60.2, M60.8, M60.9, M79.0, M79.1, M79.3, M79.6, R25.2*

incl: fibromyalgia, fibrositis, myalgia, panniculitis, rheumatism
excl: pain in spine L01, L02, L03; leg cramps L14

L19 Muscle symptom/complaint NOS   *M62.5, M62.6, M79.9*

incl: atrophy/wasting/weakness of muscle, muscle stiffness/strain
excl: pain in spine L01, L02, L03; leg cramps L14; 'growing pains' in child L29;
            restless legs N04

L20 Joint symptom/complaint NOS   *M25.4 to M25.6, M25.8, M25.9*

incl: arthralgia, effusion/swelling of joint, pain/stiffness/weakness in joint
excl: symptoms/complaints specified in L07, L08, L10–13, L15–17

L26 Fear of cancer, musculoskeletal   *Z71.1*

excl: if the patient has the disease, code the disease
criteria: concern about/fear of cancer of musculoskeletal system in a patient without
              cancer/until the diagnosis is proven

L27 Fear of musculoskeletal disease, other   *Z71.1*

excl: fear of musculoskeletal cancer L26; if the patient has the disease, code the
              disease
criteria: concern about/fear of a musculoskeletal disease in a patient without the
              disease/until the diagnosis is proven

L28 Limited function/disability (L)   *Z73.6*

excl: falls A29; limping/walking difficulties/gait problems N29
criteria: limitation of function/disability due to a musculoskeletal problem
Note: The COOP/WONCA Charts are suitable for documenting the patient's functional
status (see Chapter 8).

L29 Musculoskeletal symptom/complaint, other   *R26.8, R29.3, R29.8*

incl: 'growing pains' in a child
excl: clubbing of fingernails S22

Component 7—Diagnosis/disease

L70 Infection of musculoskeletal system
                    M00, M01, M46.2 to M46.5, M60.0, M65.0,
                    M65.1, M71.0, M71.1, M86

incl: infective tenosynovitis, osteomyelitis, pyogenic arthritis
excl: Reiter's disease L99; late effect of polio N70
criteria: infection localized in musculoskeletal system

L71 Malignant neoplasm musculoskeletal   C40, C41, C46.1, C49

incl: fibrosarcoma, osteosarcoma
excl: secondary neoplasms (code to original site), benign/unspecified musculo-
             skeletal neoplasm L97
criteria: characteristic histological appearance

L72 Fracture: radius/ulna   S52

incl: Colles' fracture
excl: pathological fracture L95, L99; non-union L99
criteria: imaging evidence of a fracture; or trauma plus visible/palpable deformity or
             crepitus involving the bone
consider: arm symptom L09; musculoskeletal injury NOS L81

L73 Fracture: tibia/fibula   S82.1 to S82.9

incl: Pott's fracture
excl: fracture patella L76; pathological fracture L95, L99; non-union L99
criteria: imaging evidence of a fracture; or trauma plus visible/palpable deformity or
             crepitus involving the bone
consider: leg symptom L14; ankle symptom L16; musculoskeletal injury NOS L81

L74 Fracture: hand/foot bone   S62, S92

incl: fracture carpal/metacarpal bone, fracture phalange hand/foot, fracture
             tarsal/metatarsal bone
excl: pathological fracture L95, L99; non-union L99
criteria: imaging evidence of a fracture; or trauma plus visible/palpable deformity or
             crepitus involving the bone
consider: arm symptom L09; leg symptom L14; musculoskeletal injury NOS L81

L75 Fracture: femur   S72

incl: fracture neck of femur
excl: pathological fracture L95, L99; non-union L99
criteria: imaging evidence of a fracture; or trauma plus visible/palpable deformity or
             crepitus involving the bone
consider: leg symptom L14; musculoskeletal injury NOS L81

L76 Fracture: other
             S02.2 to S02.4, S02.6 to S02.9, S12, S22, S32, S42, S82.0, T08, T10, T12, T14.2

excl: fractures specified in L72, L73, L74, and L75; pathological fracture L95,
             L99; non-union L99; skull fracture N80
criteria: imaging evidence of a fracture; or trauma plus visible/palpable displacement
             of the bone surface
consider: symptoms in Component 1

L77 Sprain/strain of ankle   *S93.4*

criteria: stretch injury of the affected part plus pain aggravated by stretching or tensing the affected structure
consider: ankle symptom L16

L78 Sprain/strain of knee   *S83.4, S83.6*

excl: acute damage of meniscus/internal ligament of knee L96
criteria: stretch injury of the affected part plus pain aggravated by stretching or tensing the affected structure

L79 Sprain/strain of joint NOS
S03.4, S03.5, S13.4 to S13.6, S23.3 to S23.5, S33.6, S43.4 to S43.7, S53.2 to S53.4, S63.3 to S63.7, S73.1, S93.2, S93.5, S93.6, T09.2, T11.2, T13.2, T14.3

incl: sprain/strain of other joint/ligament, whiplash
excl: sprain/strain ankle L77; sprain/strain knee L78; back strain L84
criteria: stretch injury of the affected part plus pain aggravated by stretching or tensing the affected structure
consider: symptoms in Component 1

L80 Dislocation/subluxation
M22.0, M22.1, S03.0, S03.3, S13.0 to S13.3, S23.0 to S23.2, S33.0 to S33.3, S43.0 to S43.3, S53.0, S53.1, S63.0 to S63.2, S73.0, S83.0, S83.1, S93.0, S93.1, S93.3, T09.2, T11.2, T13.2, T14.3

incl: dislocation/subluxation any site, including spine
criteria: trauma to the joint plus either imaging evidence of a dislocation/subluxation, or palpable/visible dislocation deformity
consider: symptoms in Component 1
Note: Code fracture dislocations to the fracture.

L81 Injury musculoskeletal NOS
M79.5, S09.1, S09.9, S16, S20.2, S30.0, S30.1, S33.4, S39.0, S39.8, S39.9, S40.0, S46 to S49, S50.0, S50.1, S56 to S59, S60.0 to S60.2, S66 to S69, S70.0, S70.1, S76 to S79, S80.0, S80.1, S86 to S89, S90.0 to S90.3, S96 to S99, T06.4, T09.0, T09.5 to T09.9, T11.0, T11.5 to T11.9, T13.0, T13.5 to T13.9, T14.6, T14.7

incl: deep foreign body, haemarthrosis, traumatic amputation
excl: internal injury of chest/abdomen/pelvis, multiple trauma A81; late effect trauma/deformity/disability/scarring A82; injury teeth D80; injury eardrum H77; traumatic arthropathy L91; non/mal-union of fracture L99; head injury/concussion/intracranial injury/skull fracture N80; laceration/other injury to nerve N81; insect bite/sting S12; animal bite S13; bruise/contusion S16; laceration/open wound S18

L82 Congenital anomaly musculoskeletal   *Q65 to Q79*

incl: bow leg, clubfoot (talipes), congenital dislocation of hip, genu recurvatum, con-
            genital malformation of skull and face, other congenital deformity of the foot
excl: scoliosis L85; pes planus (acquired) L98; spina bifida N85

L83 Neck syndrome

M43.0, M43.1, M43.3 to M43.6, M46.0, M47.1, M47.2, M47.8, M47.9,
M48, M50, M53.0, M53.1, M53.8, M53.9

incl: syndromes with/without radiation of pain: cervical disc lesion, cervico-
            brachial syndrome, cervicogenic headache, osteoarthritis of neck, radicular
            syndrome of upper limbs, spondylosis, torticollis

L84 Back syndrome without radiating pain

M43.0, M43.1, M43.5, M46.0, M46.1, M46.8, M46.9, M47.0, M47.8, M47.9,
M48, M51.2 to M51.9, M53.2 to M53.9, S33.5, S33.7

incl: back strain, collapsed vertebra NOS, facet joint degeneration, osteoarthrosis/
            osteoarthritis of spine, spondylolisthesis, spondylosis
excl: coccydynia L03; syndrome related to the neck L83; back pain with radiation/
            sciatica L86; psychogenic backache P75
criteria: back pain without radiation plus limitation of movement confirmed at medical
            examination
consider: symptom/complaint back L02; symptom/complaint low back L03

L85 Acquired deformity of spine   *M40, M41, M43.8, M43.9*

incl: kyphoscoliosis, kyphosis, lordosis, scoliosis
excl: congenital deformity L82; ankylosing spondylitis L88; spondylolisthesis L84

L86 Back syndrome with radiating pain   *M47.1, M47.2, M51, M54.3, M54.4*

incl: disc prolapse/degeneration, sciatica
excl: cervical disc lesion L83; spondylolisthesis L84; recent back strain L84
criteria: pain in the lumbar/thoracic region of the spine, accompanied by pain radiating
            to, or a neurological deficit of an appropriate area; or sciatica, pain radiating
            down the back of the leg, aggravated by coughing, movement, or posture; or
            demonstration of a prolapsed lumbar or thoracic disc by appropriate imaging
            technique, or at surgery
consider: back pain L02; low back pain L03
Note: Exclude referred pain that is diffuse.

L87 Bursitis/tendinitis/synovitis NOS

M65.2 to M65.4, M65.8, M65.9, M67.3, M67.4, M70, M71.2 to M71.9,
M72, M76, M77.0, M77.2, M77.3, M77.8, M77.9

incl: bone spurs, calcified tendon, Dupuytren's contracture, fasciitis, ganglion,
            synovial cysts, tenosynovitis, trigger finger   *(cont.)*

excl: bursitis/tenditis/synovitis of shoulder L92; tennis elbow/lateral epicon-
        dylitis L93

L88 Rheumatoid/seropositive arthritis   *M05, M06, M08, M45*

incl: allied conditions: ankylosing spondylitis, juvenile arthritis
excl: psoriatic arthropathy L99

L89 Osteoarthrosis of hip   *M16*

incl: osteoarthritis of hip secondary to dysplasia/trauma
criteria: either characteristic imaging appearance; or joint disorder of at least
          3 months' duration, with no constitutional symptoms and three or more of the
          following: intermittent swelling; crepitation; stiffness/limitation of move-
          ment; normal ESR, rheumatoid tests, and uric acid; over 40 years of age
consider: joint symptom L20; arthritis NOS L91

L90 Osteoarthrosis of knee   *M17*

incl: osteoarthritis of knee secondary to dysplasia/trauma
criteria: either characteristic imaging appearance; or joint disorder of at least 3
          months' duration, with no constitutional symptoms and three or more of the
          following: intermittent swelling; crepitation; stiffness/limitation of move-
          ment; normal ESR, rheumatoid tests, and uric acid; over 40 years of age
consider: joint symptom L20; arthritis NOS L91

L91 Osteoarthrosis, other   *M13, M15, M18, M19*

incl: arthritis NOS, osteoarthritis, traumatic arthropathy
excl: osteoarthrosis of neck L83; osteoarthrosis of spine L84; osteoarthrosis of
          hip L89; osteoarthrosis of knee L90; osteoarthrosis of shoulder L92
criteria: characteristic imaging appearance; or Heberden's nodes or joint disorder of
          at least 3 months' duration, with no constitutional symptoms and three or more
          of the following: intermittent swelling; crepitation; stiffness/limitation of
          movement; normal ESR, rheumatoid tests, and uric acid; over 40 years of age
consider: joint symptom L20

L92 Shoulder syndrome   *M19, M75*

incl: bursitis of shoulder, frozen shoulder, osteoarthrosis/synovitis of shoulder,
          rotator cuff syndrome, tendinitis around shoulder
criteria: shoulder pain with limitation of movement/local tenderness/crepitus; or
          periarticular calcification on imaging

L93 Tennis elbow   *M77.1*

incl: lateral epicondylitis
excl: other tendinitis L87

L94 Osteochondrosis   *M42, M91 to M93*

incl: Legg–Calvé–Perthes disease, Osgood–Schlatter disease, osteochondritis
            dissecans, Scheuermann's disease, slipped femoral epiphysis

L95 Osteoporosis   *M80 to M82*

incl: pathological fracture due to osteoporosis
criteria: characteristic imaging appearance

L96 Acute internal damage knee   *S83.2, S83.3, S83.5, S83.7*

incl: acute damage to meniscus/cruciate ligaments
excl: acute damage to collateral ligaments L78; dislocation of patella L80; chronic
            internal damage to knee L99
criteria: an initial injury that occurred no longer than 1 month previously and demon-
            stration of ligament/meniscus tear by surgery/arthroscopy/imaging, or by
            locking/giving way, pain, and swelling of knee
consider: knee symptom L15; sprain of knee L78

L97 Neoplasm musculoskeletal benign/unspecified   *D16, D21, D48.0, D48.1*

incl: benign musculoskeletal neoplasm, musculoskeletal neoplasm not specified
            as benign or malignant/when histology is not available
excl: malignant musculoskeletal neoplasm L71

L98 Acquired deformity of limb   *M20, M21*

incl: bunion, genu valgum-varum, hallux valgus/varus, mallet finger, pes planus
            (flatfoot)
excl: general congenital deformity/anomaly A90; musculoskeletal genital deformity/
            anomaly L82

L99 Musculoskeletal disease, other
M02, M03, M07, M09, M12, M14, M22.2 to M22.9, M23, M24, M25.0 to
M25.3, M25.7 to M25.9, M32 to M36, M43.2, M49, M54.1, M61,
M62.0 to M62.4, M62.8, M62.9, M63, M66, M67.0 to M67.2,
M67.8, M67.9, M68, M73, M79.4, M79.8, M84, M85,
M87 to M90, M94, M95, M99, T79.6, Z89, Z98.1

incl: arthrodesis, chronic internal derangement of knee, contractures, costochondritis,
            dermatomyositis, disorder of patella, mal-union/non-union of fracture, myositis,
            Paget's disease of bone, pathological fracture NOS, polymyalgia rheumatica,
            psoriatic arthritis (code also S91), Reiter's disease, scleroderma, Sjögren's
            syndrome, spontaneous rupture tendon, systemic lupus erythematosus
excl: hyperuricaemia A91; pathological fracture due to osteoporosis L95; post-
            polio paralysis N70; post-stroke paralysis N81; gout T92; pseudogout/crystal
            arthropathy, osteomalacia T99

N Neurological

Component 1—Symptoms and complaints

N01 Headache   *G44.3, G44.8, R51*

incl: post-traumatic headache
excl: cervicogenic headache L83; face pain N03; migraine N89; cluster headache
            N90; tension headache N95; atypical facial neuralgia N99; sinus pain R09;
            post-herpetic pain S70

N03 Pain, face   *G50.1, R51*

excl: toothache D19; headache N01; migraine N89; trigeminal neuralgia N92;
            sinus pain R09; post-herpetic pain S70

N04 Restless legs   *G25.8*

excl: leg cramps L14; intermittent claudication K92

N05 Tingling fingers/feet/toes   *R20.2*

incl: burning sensation, prickly feeling fingers/feet/toes, paraesthesia
excl: pain/tenderness of skin S01

N06 Sensation disturbance, other   *R20.0, R20.1, R20.3, R20.8*

incl: anaesthesia, numbness
excl: tingling fingers/feet/toes N05; pain/tenderness of skin S01

N07 Convulsion/seizure   *R56*

incl: febrile convulsion, fit
excl: fainting A06; transient ischaemic attack K89

N08 Abnormal involuntary movements   *G25, R25.0, R25.1, R25.3, R25.8, R29.0*

incl: dystonic movements, jerking, myoclonus, shaking, tetany, tremor, twitching
excl: chorea K71; cramps/spasm L07, L09, L12, L14, L17, L18; restless legs
            N04; convulsion N07; tic douloureux N92; dystonia/organic tic N99;
            psychogenic tic P10

N16 Disturbance of smell/taste   *R43*

incl: anosmia
excl: halitosis D20

N17 Vertigo/dizziness   *R42*

incl: giddiness, feeling faint/lightheaded, loss of balance, woozy
excl: syncope/blackout A06; motion sickness A88; specific vertiginous syndrome H82

N18 Paralysis/weakness   *G98*

incl: paresis
excl: general weakness A04

N19 Speech disorder   *R47*

incl: aphasia, dysphasia, dysarthria, slurred speech
excl: stammering/stuttering P10; speech delay P22; hoarseness R23

N26 Fear of cancer of neurological system   *Z71.1*

excl: if the patient has the disease, code the disease
criteria: concern about/fear of neurological cancer in a patient without the disease/
             until the diagnosis is proven

N27 Fear of neurological disease, other   *Z71.1*

excl: fear of neurological cancer N26; if the patient has the disease, code the disease
criteria: concern about/fear of other neurological disease in a patient without the
             disease/until the diagnosis is proven

N28 Limited function/disability (N)   *Z73.6*

incl: disability due to neurological diseases and disorders
criteria: limitation of function/disability due to a neurological problem
Note: The COOP/WONCA Charts are suitable for documenting the patient's functional
status (see Chapter 8).

N29 Neurological symptom/complaint, other

M79.2, R26, R27, R29.0 to R29.2, R29.8

incl: ataxia, gait abnormality, limping, meningism

Component 7—Diagnosis/diseases

N70 Poliomyelitis   *A80, A85.0, B91*

incl: late effect of poliomyelitis, post-polio syndrome, other neurological
             enterovirus infection

N71 Meningitis/encephalitis
> *A32.1, A39.0, A83, A84, A85.1, A85.2, A85.8, A86, A87, B00.3, B00.4,*
> *B37.5, B58.2, B94.1, G00 to G05*

criteria: an acute febrile illness with abnormal findings in the cerebrospinal fluid
consider: fever A03; meningism N29

N72 Tetanus
A33 to A35

excl: tetany N08
criteria: rigidity, hypertonic contractions or tetanic spasticity and a history of preceding injury

N73 Neurological infection, other
A81, A88.8, A89, G06 to G09

incl: cerebral abscess, slow virus infection
excl: poliomyelitis N70; meningitis/encephalitis N71; acute polyneuritis N94

N74 Malignant neoplasm nervous system
C47, C70 to C72

criteria: characteristic histological appearance
consider: unspecified neoplasm nervous system N76

N75 Benign neoplasm nervous system
D32, D33, D36.1

incl: acoustic neuroma, meningioma

N76 Neoplasm nervous system, unspecified
D42, D43, D48.2

incl: neoplasm nervous system not specified as benign or malignant/when histology is not available
excl: neurofibromatosis A90

N79 Concussion
S06.0

incl: late effect of concussion
excl: psychological effect of concussion P02
criteria: trauma to the head with a temporary loss of consciousness and/or neurological sequela
consider: other head injury N80

N80 Head injury, other
> *S02.0, S02.1, S02.9, S06.1 to S06.9, S07, S08.0, S08.8, S08.9, S09.0, S09.7 to S09.9*

incl: cerebral contusion, cerebral injury with/without skull fracture, extradural haematoma, subdural haematoma, traumatic intracranial haemorrhage *(cont.)*

excl: concussion N79
criteria: trauma to the head, complicated by cerebral damage

N81 Injury nervous system, other
> *S04, S09.9, S14, S24, S34, S44, S54, S64, S74, S84, S94, T06.0 to T06.2,*
> *T09.3, T09.4, T11.3, T13.3, T14.4*

incl: nerve injury, spinal cord injury

N85 Congenital anomaly neurological   *Q00 to Q07*

incl: hydrocephalus, spina bifida

N86 Multiple sclerosis   *G35*

incl: disseminated sclerosis
criteria: exacerbations/remissions of multiple neurological manifestation with
             deficits/derangements disseminated in both time and site (any combination
             of neurological signs and symptoms is possible)
consider: other neurological symptom N29

N87 Parkinsonism   *G20 to G22*

incl: drug-induced parkinsonism, paralysis agitans, Parkinson's disease
criteria: poverty and slowness of voluntary movements, resting tremor improving
             with active purposeful movement, and muscular rigidity
consider: abnormal involuntary movements N08; disorder of speech N19

N88 Epilepsy   *G40, G41*

incl: all types of epilepsy: focal seizures, generalized seizures, grand mal, petit mal,
             status epilepticus
criteria: recurrent episodes of sudden altered consciousness, with/without
             tonic/clonic movements/seizure, plus either eyewitness account of the attack,
             or characteristic abnormality of electroencephalogram (EEG)
consider: convulsion N07; other neurological symptom N29

N89 Migraine   *G43, G44.1*

incl: vascular headache with/without aura
excl: cervicogenic headache L83; cluster headache N90; tension headache N95
criteria: recurrent episodes of headache with three or more of the following: unilateral
             headache; nausea/vomiting; aura; other neurological symptoms; family history
             of migraine
consider: headache N01

N90 Cluster headache   *G44.0*

excl: migraine N89
criteria: attacks of severe, often excruciating unilateral pain peri-orbitally and/or temporally, occurring up to eight times a day, sometimes associated with conjunctival injection, lacrimation, nasal congestion, rhinorrhoea, sweating, miosis, ptosis, or eyelid oedema. Attacks occur in cluster periods lasting weeks/months separated by remissions lasting months/years

N91 Facial paralysis/Bell's palsy   *G51, G53*

criteria: acute onset of unilateral paralysis of muscles of facial expression without sensory loss
consider: paralysis/weakness N18

N92 Trigeminal neuralgia   *G50.0, G50.8, G50.9*

incl: tic douloureux
excl: post-herpetic neuralgia S70
criteria: unilateral paroxysms of burning facial pain aggravated by touching trigger-points, blowing nose or yawning, without sensory or motor paralysis
consider: neuralgia NOS N99

N93 Carpal tunnel syndrome   *G56.0*

criteria: loss/impairment of superficial sensation affecting the thumb, index and middle finger, that may or may not split the ring finger. Dysaesthesia and pain worsen usually during the night, and may radiate to the forearm
consider: sensation disturbance N06

N94 Peripheral neuritis/neuropathy
G54, G55, G56.1 to G56.4, G56.8, G56.9, G57 to G64, M79.2

incl: acute infective polyneuropathy, diabetic neuropathy (double code with T89, T90), Guillain–Barré syndrome, nerve lesion, neuropathy, phantom limb
excl: post-herpetic neuropathy S70
criteria: sensory, reflex and motor changes confined to the territory of individual nerves, sometimes without apparent cause, sometimes secondary to a specific disease, e.g. diabetes

N95 Tension headache   *G44.2*

excl: migraine N89; cluster headache N90
criteria: pressing, generalized headache associated with stress and muscle tension with/without increased tenderness of pericranial muscles
consider: headache N01

N99 Neurological disease, other

> *E51.2, G10 to G13, G23, G24, G26, G31.0, G31.1, G31.8, G31.9, G32, G36, G37, G52, G70 to G73, G80 to G83, G90 to G92, G93.0 to G93.2, G93.4 to G93.9, G94 to G96, G98, G99, M79.2, Z98.2*

incl: cerebral palsy, dystonia, motor neuron disease, myasthenia gravis, neuralgia NOS

excl: sleep apnoea P06

P Psychological

Component 1—Symptoms and complaints

P01 Feeling anxious/nervous/tense   *R45.0*

incl: anxiety NOS, feeling frightened
excl: anxiety disorder P74
criteria: feelings reported by the patient as an emotional or psychological experience not attributed to the presence of a mental disorder. A gradual transition exists from feelings that are unwelcome, but quite normal, and feelings that are so troublesome to the patient that professional help is sought

P02 Acute stress reaction   *F43.0, F43.2, F43.8, F43.9*

incl: adjustment disorder, culture shock, feeling stressed/grief/homesick, immediate post-traumatic stress, shock (psychic)
excl: feeling depressed P03; depressive disorder P76; post-traumatic stress disorder P82
criteria: a reaction to a stressful life event or significant life change requiring a major adjustment, either as an expected response to the event or as a maladaptive response interfering with daily coping and resulting in impaired social functioning, with recovery within a limited period of time

P03 Feeling depressed   *R45.2, R45.3*

incl: feeling inadequate, unhappy, worried
excl: low self-esteem P28; depressive disorder P76
criteria: feelings reported by the patient as an emotional or psychological experience not attributed to the presence of a mental disorder. A gradual transition exists from feelings that are unwelcome, but quite normal, and feelings that are so troublesome to the patient that professional help is sought

P04 Feeling/behaving irritable/angry   *R45.1, R45.4 to R45.6*

incl: agitation NOS, restlessness NOS
excl: overactive child P22; irritability in partner Z13   *(cont.)*

criteria: feelings reported by the patient as an emotional or psychological experience not attributed to the presence of a mental disorder, or behaviour indicating irritability or anger. A gradual transition exists from feelings or behaviour that are unwelcome, but quite normal, to those that are so troublesome that professional help is sought

P05 Senility, feeling/behaving old *R54*

incl: concern with aging, senescence
excl: dementia P70
criteria: feelings reported by the patient as an emotional or psychological experience not attributed to the presence of a mental disorder. A gradual transition exists from feelings that are unwelcome, but quite normal, to feelings that are so troublesome to the patient that professional help is sought

P06 Sleep disturbance *F51, G47*

incl: insomnia, nightmares, sleep apnoea, sleepwalking, somnolence
excl: jetlag A88
criteria: sleep disturbance as a diagnosis requires that the sleeping problem forms a major complaint that, according to both patient and doctor, is not caused by another disorder but is a condition in its own right. Insomnia requires a quantitative or qualitative deficiency of sleep that is unsatisfactory, in the patient's opinion, over a considerable period of time. In hypersomnia excessive daytime sleepiness and sleep attacks exist that limit the patient's performance

P07 Sexual desire reduced *F52.0*

incl: frigidity, loss of libido
excl: non-organic impotence/loss of sexual fulfilment P08; concern with sexual preference P09
criteria: sexual problems with regard to desire not caused by any organic disorder or disease, but a reflection of the inability of a patient to participate in the sexual relationship s/he wants because of lack of desire, failure of genital response or function

P08 Sexual fulfilment reduced *F52.1 to F52.9*

incl: non-organic impotence or dyspareunia, premature ejaculation, vaginismus of psychogenic origin
excl: sexual problems with desire P07; concern with sexual preference P09; vaginismus NOS X04; organic impotence/sexual problems Y07
criteria: sexual problems with regard to fulfilment not caused by any organic disorder or disease, but a reflection of the inability of a patient to participate in the sexual relationship s/he wants because of failure of genital response or function, or problems with sexual development

P09 Sexual preference concern   *F64 to F66*

excl: reduced sexual desire P07; reduced sexual fulfilment P08
criteria: sexual problems with regard to preference not caused by any organic disorder
            or disease, but a reflection of the inability of a patient to participate in the
            sexual relationship s/he wants because of problems with sexual identity,
            preference or orientation

P10 Stammering/stuttering/tic   *F95, F98.4 to F98.6*

excl: tic douloureux N92
criteria: stammering and stuttering: disorder of speech characterized by frequent rep-
            etitions/prolongations of sounds, or by frequent hesitations/pauses
            disrupting speech

P11 Eating problem in child   *F98.2, F98.3*

incl: feeding problem, problem with eating behaviour of child
excl: anorexia nervosa P86; eating problem in adult T05
Note: Behavioural problems in children are particularly difficult to classify, as illustrated
by the fact that they are distributed over four chapters of ICPC. Whether or not parents
present these problems to a GP will reflect their ideas about the gradual differences
between normal (though perhaps annoying) behaviour and behaviour that is considered
worrying or 'pathological'.

P12 Bedwetting/enuresis   *F98.0*

excl: bedwetting due to organic disorder U04
criteria: involuntary voiding of urine by day/night not determined to be related to any
            organic disorder
Note: Behavioural problems in children are particularly difficult to classify, as illustrated
by the fact that they are distributed over four chapters of ICPC. Whether or not parents
present these problems to a GP will reflect their ideas about the gradual differences
between normal (though perhaps annoying) behaviour and behaviour that is considered
worrying or 'pathological'.

P13 Encopresis/bowel training problem   *F98.1*

criteria: encopresis requires repeated passage of usually well formed faeces in inap-
            propriate places, considered abnormal in relation to age, and not caused by
            constipation/sphincter control disorder/another disease

P15 Chronic alcohol abuse   *F10.1 to F10.9, G31.2*

incl: alcohol brain syndrome, alcohol psychosis, alcoholism, delirium tremens
criteria: a disorder due to the use of alcohol resulting in one or more of the following:
            harmful use with clinically important damage to health; dependence syn-
            drome; withdrawal state; psychotic disorder   *(cont.)*

Note: Substance abuse problem definitions should take into account the considerable differences between countries and cultures. A doctor can decide to label an episode as 'chronic alcohol abuse' without the patient's agreement, and consequently also without the patient's willingness to agree to any medical intervention.

P16 Acute alcohol abuse   *F10.0*

incl: drunk
criteria: a disorder due to the use of alcohol resulting in acute intoxication, with/without
             a background of chronic abuse
Note: A doctor can decide to label an episode as 'acute alcohol abuse' without the patient's agreement, and consequently also without the patient's willingness to agree to any medical intervention.

P17 Tobacco abuse   *F17*

incl: smoking problem
criteria: a disorder due to the use of tobacco resulting in one or more of the follow-
             ing: acute intoxication; harmful use with clinically important damage to
             health; dependence syndrome; withdrawal state
consider: risk factor NOS A23
Note: Substance abuse problem definitions should take into account the considerable differences between countries and cultures. An alcohol-dependent or heroin-addicted patient needs medical attention, but the definitions of 'tobacco abuse' are controversial. A physician can decide to label an episode as 'tobacco abuse' without the patient's agreement, and consequently also without the patient's willingness to agree to any medical intervention.

P18 Medication abuse   *F13, F19, F55*

incl: abuse of any prescribed drug
Note: Substance abuse problem definitions should take into account the considerable differences between countries and cultures. Some patients request and use tranquilliz-ers, sleeping tablets, anorectics, or laxatives inappropriately and for too long. In these cases physicians can decide to label the episode as 'medicine abuse' without the patient's agreement, and consequently also without the patient's willingness to agree to any medical intervention.

P19 Drug abuse   *F11 to F16, F18, F19*

incl: addiction to drug, drug withdrawal
criteria: a disorder due to the use of a dependence-producing psychoactive substance,
             resulting in one or more of the following conditions:
             acute intoxication;
             harmful use with clinically important damage to health;
             dependence syndrome;

(cont.)

withdrawal state;
        psychotic disorder;
Note: Substance abuse problem definitions should take into account the considerable differences between countries and cultures. An alcohol-dependent or heroin-addicted patient needs medical attention, but the definitions of 'use of hashish' are controversial. Doctors can decide to label an episode as 'drug abuse' without the patient's agreement, and consequently also without the patient's willingness to agree to any medical intervention.

P20 Memory disturbance   *R41*

incl: amnesia, disorientation, disturbance of concentration

P22 Child behaviour symptom/complaint

F91 to F94, F98.8, F98.9, R62.0

incl: delayed milestones, jealousy, overactive child, speech delay, temper tantrum
excl: behaviour symptom/complaint adolescent, adult P23, P80; concern about
            physical development/growth delay T10

P23 Adolescent behaviour symptom/complaint   *F91, F92, F94, F98.8, F98.9*

incl: delinquency
excl: behaviour symptom/complaint child, adult P22, P80, P81

P24 Specific learning problem   *F80 to F83, R48*

incl: dyslexia
excl: attention deficit disorder P81; mental retardation P85
criteria: specific speech, language and learning problems with onset in childhood,
            together with an impairment of functions related to biological maturation of
            the central nervous system, and a steady course over time without sponta-
            neous remissions or relapses, although the deficit may diminish as the child
            grows older

P25 Phase of life problem, adult   *Z60.0*

incl: empty nest syndrome, mid-life crisis, retirement problem
excl: senility, feeling/behaving old P05; menopause X11

P27 Fear of mental disorder   *Z71.1*

incl: concern about mental disease, fear of attempting suicide
excl: if the patient has the disease, code the disease
criteria: concern about/fear of mental disease in a patient without the disease/until
            the diagnosis is proven

P28 Limited function/disability (P) *Z73.6*

incl: low self-esteem
criteria: limitation of function/disability due to a psychological problem
Note: The COOP/WONCA Charts are suitable for documenting the patient's functional
status (see Chapter 8).

P29 Psychological symptom/complaint, other

F50.8, F50.9, F63.3, F98.8, F98.9, R44, R45.7, R45.8, R46
Z64.2, Z64.3, Z73.0, Z73.1, Z73.3

incl: delusions, eating disorders NOS, hallucinations, multiple psychological
symptoms/complaints, poor hygiene, strange behaviour, suspiciousness
excl: tension headache N95

Component 7—Diagnosis/diseases

Note: A mental disorder is a clinically significant psychological syndrome or
pattern, with or without an association with stressors (such as disability, increased
risk, or an important loss), that cannot be considered an expected response to a particular event, but rather a manifestation of a behavioural, psychological, or biological
dysfunction.

P70 Dementia *F00 to F03, G30*

incl: Alzheimer's disease, senile dementia
criteria: a syndrome due to a disease of the brain, usually of a chronic and/or pro-
gressive nature, with clinically significant disturbance of multiple higher
cortical functions (memory, thinking, orientation, comprehension), together
with intact consciousness
consider: senility P05; other psychological symptoms P29

P71 Organic psychosis, other *F04 to F07, F09*

incl: delirium
excl: psychosis caused by alcohol P15; psychosis NOS P98
criteria: organic psychiatric disorders as a diagnosis require psychological syndromes,
patterns or behaviour due to organic disease

P72 Schizophrenia *F20 to F22, F24, F25, F28*

incl: all types of schizophrenia, paranoia
excl: acute/transient psychosis P98
criteria: fundamental and characteristic distortions of thinking, perception, and affect
that are inappropriate or blunted (e.g. thought-echo, -insertion, -withdrawal,

(cont.)

delusional perceptions, hallucinatory voices, delusions of control), together
with a clear consciousness and unaffected intellectual capacity
consider: psychosis NOS P98

P73 Affective psychosis   *F30, F31, F34.0*

incl: bipolar disorder, hypomania, mania, manic depression
excl: depression P76
criteria: a fundamental disturbance in affect and mood, alternately being elated and
              depressed (with/without associated anxiety). In manic disorder mood, energy,
              and activity are simultaneously elevated. In bipolar disease, at least two periods
              of disturbed mood, shifting from elevated to lowered, are observed
consider: psychosis NOS P98

P74 Anxiety disorder/anxiety state   *F41.0, F41.1, F41.3 to F41.9*

incl: anxiety neurosis, panic disorder
excl: anxiety with depression P76; anxiety NOS P01
criteria: clinically significant anxiety that is not restricted to any particular environ-
              mental situation. It manifests as a panic disorder (recurrent attacks of severe
              anxiety not restricted to any particular situation, with/without physical
              symptoms) or as a disorder in which generalized and persistent anxiety, not
              related to any particular situation, occurs with variable physical symptoms
consider: feeling anxious/nervous/tense P01

P75 Somatization disorder   *F44, F45.0 to F45.2*

incl: conversion disorder, hypochondriacal disorder, hysteria, pseudocyesis
criteria: somatization disorder is characterized by a preoccupation with and repeated
              presentations of physical symptoms and complaints together with persistent
              requests for medical investigations in spite of repeated negative findings and
              reassurances by doctors. For this diagnosis, the presentation of multiple,
              recurrent, and frequently changing physical symptoms presented to the family
              physician over a period of at least 1 year is required. Hypochondriacal disorder
              requires a persistent preoccupation with either the physical appearance or
              with the possibility of having a serious disease, together with persistent somatic
              complaints over a period of at least 1 year, in spite of repeated negative findings
              and reassurances by doctors
Note: Somatization is the repeated presentation of physical symptoms and complaints
suggesting physical disorders for which no demonstrable organic findings or physiological mechanisms are responsible, and for which there is positive evidence that they are
linked to psychological factors, while the patient does not experience a sense of con-
trolling the production of these symptoms in dealing with the psychological factors.
Physical symptoms and complaints including pain that are presented as if they were due
to a physical disorder of a system/organ under autonomic nervous control, or that consist
of persistent, severe/distressing pain that cannot be explained by a physiological
(cont.)

process/disorder, are coded with a symptom/complaint diagnosis representing the physical aspect, and—if possible—with a code representing the emotional or psychosocial problem with which it is associated.

The definition of somatization disorder in ICD-10 (a minimum of 2 years) is too stringent for use in general practice.

P76 Depressive disorder   *F32, F33, F34.1, F34.8, F34.9, F38, F39, F41.2, F53.0*

incl: depressive neurosis/psychosis, mixed anxiety and depression, reactive depression, puerperal/postnatal depression

excl: acute stress reaction P02

criteria: fundamental disturbance in affect and mood towards depression. Mood, energy and activity are simultaneously lowered, together with an impaired capacity for enjoyment, interest, and concentration. Sleep and appetite are usually disturbed, and self-esteem and confidence are decreased

consider: feeling depressed P03

P77 Suicide/suicide attempt   *Z91.5*

incl: suicide gesture, successful attempt (double code with A96)

excl: fear of committing suicide P27

P78 Neuraesthenia, surmenage   *F48.0*

criteria: increased fatiguability with unpleasant associations, difficulties in concentration, and a persistent decrease in performance and coping efficiency; the feeling of physical weakness and exhaustion after mental effort or after a minimal physical effort is often accompanied by muscular pain and an inability to relax

consider: fatigue/postviral fatigue/chronic fatigue syndrome A04

P79 Phobia/compulsive disorder   *F40, F42*

criteria: phobic anxiety disorder requires outspoken anxiety, evoked only in well defined situations that are not generally considered dangerous; the patient tries to avoid these situations, or endures them with dread.
Obsessive compulsive disorder requires distressing and recurrent obsessional thoughts/acts recognized by the patient as his/her own; compulsive stereotyped behaviours are repeated again and again, intended to prevent some objective, unlikely event and recognized by the patient as pointless and ineffective

P80 Personality disorder   *F60 to F62, F63.0 to F63.2, F63.8, F63.9, F68, F69*

incl: psychopathy, compensation neurosis, Munchausen's syndrome, adult behaviour disorder

criteria: persistent and clinically important conditions and behaviour patterns in an individual's lifestyle and mode of relating to him/herself and others, reflecting

(cont.)

significant/extreme deviations from the way an average individual in a given culture perceives, feels, and behaves. This pattern is deeply ingrained and longlasting

P81 Hyperkinetic disorder   *F90*

incl: attention deficit disorder (ADD), hyperactivity
excl: hyperkinetic disorder with adolescent onset P23; learning disorder P24
criteria: early onset of a lack of persistence in activities requiring cognitive involve-
            ment, with a tendency to move from one activity to another without completing
            any one, with disorganized and ill regulated behaviour, and excessive activity
consider: overactive child P22

P82 Post-traumatic stress disorder   *F43.1*

incl: persistent adjustment disorder
criteria: a stressful event followed by a major state of distress and disturbance, with a
            delayed or protracted reaction, flashbacks, nightmares, emotional blunting, and
            anhedonia interfering with social functioning and performance, and including
            depressed mood, anxiety, worry, and feeling unable to cope, persistent over time
consider: feeling anxious P01; acute stress reaction P02; feeling depressed P03

P85 Mental retardation   *F70 to F73, F78, F79*

excl: mental retardation due to congenital anomaly A90
criteria: arrested/incomplete development of the mind with impairment of skills during
            the developmental period, and a low overall level of intelligence, with/without
            impairment of behaviour

P86 Anorexia nervosa/bulimia   *F50.0 to F50.4*

criteria: *Anorexia nervosa*: deliberate weight loss induced and sustained by the
            patient, associated with an intensive and overvalued dread of fatness and
            flabbiness of body contours;
            Bulimia: repeated bouts of overeating and an excessive preoccupation with
            bodyweight, leading to a pattern of overeating followed by induced vomiting
            or use of purgatives
consider: eating disorder, food refusal P11, P29; feeding problem T04, T05

P98 Psychosis NOS, other   *F23, F29, F53.1*

incl: acute/transient/reactive/puerperal psychosis

P99 Psychological disorders, other
                    F48.1, F48.8, F48.9, F53.8, F53.9, F54, F59, F84, F88, F89, F99

incl: autism, neurosis NOS

R Respiratory

Component 1—Symptoms and complaints

R01 Pain, respiratory system *R07.1*

incl: painful respiration, pleuritic pain, pleurodynia
excl: chest pain A11; musculoskeletal chest pain L04; nose pain R08; sinus pain R09; sore throat R21; chest tightness R29; pleurisy R82

R02 Shortness of breath/dyspnoea *R06.0*

incl: orthopnoea
excl: wheezing R03; stridor R04; hyperventilation R98

R03 Wheezing *R06.2*

incl: inspiratory wheeze, rhonchi
excl: dyspnoea R02; stridor R04; hyperventilation R98

R04 Breathing problem, other *R06.1, R06.3, R06.5, R06.8*

incl: abnormal breathing, apnoea, holding breath, respiratory distress, snoring, stridor, tachypnoea
excl: sleep apnoea P06; respiratory pain R01; dyspnoea R02; wheezing R03; cough R05; hyperventilation R98

R05 Cough *R05*

incl: cough (dry or moist)
excl: abnormal sputum/phlegm R25

R06 Nose bleed/epistaxis *R04.0*

R07 Sneezing/nasal congestion *J34.8, R06.7*

incl: blocked nose, rhinorrhoea, running nose

R08 Nose symptom/complaint, other *J34.8*

incl: pain in nose, postnasal drip, prominent nose, red nose
excl: anosmia N16; epistaxis R06; blocked nose/sneezing R07; complaints of sinuses R09; rhinophyma S99

R09 Sinus symptom/complaint *J34.8*

incl: blocked sinus, congested sinus, pain/pressure in sinus
excl: headache N01; face pain N03; nasal congestion R07

R21 Throat symptom/complaint   *R07.0, R09.8*

incl: dry/inflamed/red/sore throat, large tonsils, lump in throat, tonsillar pain
excl: voice symptom R23; tonsillar hypertrophy R90

R23 Voice symptom/complaint   *R49*

incl: absence of voice, aphonia, hoarseness
excl: neurological disorder of speech N19; stammering/stuttering/tic P10; sore
           throat R21

R24 Haemoptysis   *R04.2*

incl: coughing blood

R25 Sputum/phlegm abnormal   *R09.3*

excl: cough with sputum R05; haemoptysis R24

R26 Fear of cancer of respiratory system   *Z71.1*

excl: if the patient has the disease, code the disease
criteria: concern about/fear of cancer of respiratory system in a patient without the
              disease/until the diagnosis is proven

R27 Fear of respiratory disease, other   *Z71.1*

excl: fear of respiratory cancer R26; if the patient has the disease, code the disease
criteria: concern about/fear of other respiratory disease in a patient without the disease/
              until the diagnosis is proven

R28 Limited function/disability (R)   *Z73.6, Z99.1*

incl: disability due to hypoxia, hypercapnia, reduced lung function, respiratory
           disease, disease of nose/larynx/throat
excl: dyspnoea R02; wheezing R03
Note: The COOP/WONCA Charts are suitable for documenting the patient's functional
status (see Chapter 8).

R29 Respiratory symptom/complaint, other
R04.1, R04.8, R04.9, R06.6, R09.0, R09.2, R09.8

incl: chest tightness, fluid on lung, hiccough, lung congestion

Component 7—Diagnosis/diseases

R71 Whooping cough   *A37*

incl: parapertussis, pertussis
excl: croup R77
criteria: respiratory infection with a characteristic staccato paroxysmal cough ending
            with a high-pitched inspiratory whoop; or respiratory infection with cough
            of at least 3 weeks' duration in contact with known pertussis; or demonstra-
            tion of *Bordetella pertussis* or *parapertussis*
consider: cough R05; upper respiratory infection R74

R72 Strep throat   *J02.0, J03.0*

incl: proven streptococcal pharyngitis/tonsillitis
excl: scarlet fever A78; erysipelas/strep skin infection S76
criteria: acute inflammation of the throat, plus demonstration of beta-haemolytic
            streptococci
consider: tonsillitis R76

R73 Boil/abscess nose   *J34.0*

incl: localized nose infection
excl: acute sinusitis R75

R74 Upper respiratory infection, acute   *B00.2, B08.5, J00, J02.8, J02.9, J06*

incl: acute rhinitis, coryza, head cold, nasopharyngitis, pharyngitis, URTI/URI
excl: measles A71; infectious mononucleosis A75; viral pharyngoconjunctivitis
            F70; sinusitis R75; tonsillitis/quinsy R76; laryngitis/croup R77; influenza
            R80; chronic pharyngitis R83; allergic rhinitis R97
criteria: evidence of acute inflammation of nasal or pharyngeal mucosa with absence
            of criteria for more specifically defined acute respiratory infection classified
            in this section

R75 Sinusitis acute/chronic   *J01, J32*

incl: sinusitis affecting any paranasal sinus
criteria: purulent nasal/postnasal discharge, or previous medically treated episodes
            of sinusitis, plus tenderness over one/more sinuses, or deep-seated
            aching facial pain aggravated by dependency of head, or opacity on
            transillumination; or imaging evidence of sinusitis; or pus obtained from
            the sinus
consider: headache N01; face pain N03; upper respiratory tract infection R74

R76 Tonsillitis, acute   *J03.8, J03.9, J36*

incl: peritonsillar abscess, quinsy
excl: infectious mononucleosis A75; strep throat R72; diphtheria R83; hypertrophy/
              chronic infection of tonsils R90
criteria: sore throat or fever with reddening of tonsil(s) more than the posterior
              pharyngeal wall, and either pus on swollen tonsil(s) or enlarged tender
              regional lymph nodes
consider: acute upper respiratory tract infection R74

R77 Laryngitis/tracheitis, acute   *J04, J05.0*

incl: croup
excl: laryngotracheobronchitis R78; epiglottitis R83
criteria: hoarseness/stridor with/without respiratory distress, or deep dry painful
              cough (barking in children), and normal chest signs
consider: upper respiratory tract infection R74

R78 Acute bronchitis/bronchiolitis   *J20 to J22, J40*

incl: acute lower respiratory infection NOS, bronchitis NOS, chest infection
              NOS, laryngotracheobronchitis, tracheobronchitis
excl: influenza R80; chronic bronchitis R79; allergic bronchitis R96
criteria: in children and adults: cough and fever with scattered or generalized abnor-
              mal chest signs: wheeze, coarse rales, rhonchi or moist sounds; in infants
              (bronchiolitis): dyspnoea and hyperinflation
consider: wheezing R03; cough R05; upper respiratory tract infection R74

R79 Chronic bronchitis   *J41, J42*

excl: emphysema/chronic obstructive pulmonary (lung, airways) disease R95;
              bronchiectasis R99
criteria: cough with sputum on most days for at least 3 months in each of at least
              2 years; and scattered rales/rhonchi on auscultation of the chest during these
              episodes
consider: cough R05; abnormal sputum/phlegm R25; bronchitis NOS R78

R80 Influenza   *J10.1, J10.8, J11.1, J11.8*

incl: influenza-like illness, para-influenza
excl: gastric flu D70; influenza pneumonia R81
criteria: myalgia and cough without abnormal respiratory physical signs other than
              inflammation of nasal mucous membrane and throat, plus three or more of
              the following: sudden onset (within 12 h); rigors/chills/fever; prostration and
              weakness; influenza in close contacts; influenza epidemic; or viral
              culture/serological evidence of influenza virus infection
consider: fever A03; virus infection NOS A77; upper respiratory tract infection R74

R81 Pneumonia   *A48.1, J10.0, J11.0, J12 to J18*

incl: bacterial/viral pneumonia, bronchopneumonia, influenzal pneumonia,
            Legionnaire's disease, pneumonitis
excl: aspiration pneumonia R99
criteria: evidence of pulmonary consolidation
consider: cough R05; acute bronchitis R78

R82 Pleurisy/pleural effusion   *J90, J91, J94, R09.1*

incl: pleural inflammatory exudate, pleuritis
excl: tuberculosis R70; pneumonia R81; malignant effusion to be coded to origin
            of malignancy
criteria: clinical evidence of pleural exudate; or pleuritic pain accompanied by
            pleural friction rub; or investigative evidence of inflammatory pleural
            exudate
consider: pleuritic pain R01

R83 Respiratory infection, other
A36, B37.1, B44, B58.3, J05.1, J31, J37, J85, J86

incl: chronic nasopharyngitis, chronic pharyngitis, chronic rhinitis NOS, diphtheria,
            empyema, epiglottitis, fungal respiratory infection, lung abscess, protozoal
            infection (without pneumonia)
excl: cystic fibrosis T99

R84 Malignant neoplasm bronchus/lung   *C33, C34*

incl: malignancy of trachea/bronchus/lung
excl: malignancy of unknown site A79; a secondary malignancy from known site
            to be coded to site
criteria: characteristic histological appearance
consider: unspecified respiratory neoplasm R92

R85 Malignant neoplasm respiratory, other
C09 to C13, C14.0, C14.2, C30.0, C31, C32, C38.4, C39, C45.0

incl: malignancy of larynx/mediastinum/nose/pharynx/pleura/sinus, mesothelioma
excl: Hodgkin's disease B72; malignancy of trachea/bronchus/lung R84
criteria: characteristic histological appearance
consider: unspecified respiratory neoplasm R92

R86 Benign neoplasm respiratory   *D14, D19*

excl: unspecified respiratory neoplasm R92; nasal polyp R99
criteria: characteristic clinical or histological appearance

R87 Foreign body nose/larynx/bronchus   *T17*

incl: foreign body in lung
excl: drowning A88; foreign body lodged in oesophagus D79; foreign body in ear
             H76; aspiration pneumonia R99
criteria: visualization of foreign body directly/endoscopically/using imaging
consider: other complaint of respiratory system R29

R88 Injury respiratory, other
S00.3, S01.2, S03.1, S09.9, S10.0, S17.0, S19.8, S27, T27, T70.1

incl: injury/trauma to nose/respiratory system
excl: drowning A88; fractured nose L76; foreign body in respiratory system R87

R89 Congenital anomaly respiratory   *Q30 to Q34*

incl: congenital abnormality of nose/pharynx/trachea/larynx/bronchi/lungs/pleura
excl: cleft lip/palate D81; cystic fibrosis T99

R90 Hypertrophy tonsils/adenoids   *J34.8, J35*

incl: chronic tonsillitis
excl: acute tonsillitis R76; allergic rhinitis R97

R92 Neoplasm respiratory, unspecified   *D02, D38*

incl: respiratory neoplasm unspecified as benign or malignant/when histology is
             not available
excl: secondary neoplasm unknown site A79; malignant respiratory neoplasm
             R84, R85; benign respiratory neoplasm R86

R95 Chronic obstructive pulmonary disease   *J43, J44*

incl: chronic obstructive airways (COAD), lung (COLD), pulmonary (COPD)
             disease, chronic airways limitation (CAL), emphysema
excl: chronic bronchitis R79; asthma R96; bronchiectasis R99; cystic fibrosis T99
criteria: objective evidence of airway obstruction, not/only partially relieved by
             bronchodilators
consider: other breathing problem R04

R96 Asthma   *J45, J46*

incl: reactive airways disease, wheezy bronchitis
excl: bronchiolitis R78; chronic bronchitis R79; emphysema R95
criteria: recurrent episodes of reversible acute bronchial obstruction with wheeze/dry
             cough; or diagnostic test meeting currently accepted criteria for asthma
consider: wheezing R03; cough R05

R97 Allergic rhinitis *J30*

incl: hay fever, nasal allergy, vasomotor rhinitis
excl: upper respiratory tract infection R74; chronic rhinitis NOS R83

R98 Hyperventilation syndrome *R06.4*

criteria: symptoms related to hyperventilation and relieved by rebreathing expired air
consider: other breathing problem R04

R99 Respiratory disease, other
J33, J34.1 to J34.3, J34.8, J38, J39, J47, J60 to J70, J80 to J82, J84, J92, J93, J96, J98, J99, Z90.2

incl: aspiration pneumonia, bronchiectasis, deviated nasal septum, lung complication of other disease, mediastinal disease, nasal polyp, other disease of larynx; pneumoconiosis, pneumothorax, pneumonitis due to allergy/chemicals/dust/fumes/mould, pulmonary collapse, respiratory failure

S Skin

Component 1—Symptoms and complaints

S01 Pain/tenderness of skin *R20.8*

incl: burning sensation, painful lesion or rash, soreness
excl: tingling fingers/feet/toes N05; other sensation disturbance N06

S02 Pruritus *L29.8, L29.9*

incl: skin irritation
excl: anogenital pruritus D05; dermatitis artefacta S99; vulval pruritus X16; nipple pruritus X20

S03 Warts *B07*

incl: verrucae
excl: molluscum contagiosum S95; genital warts X91, Y76

S04 Lump/swelling, localized *R22.0 to R22.4, R22.9, R23.8*

incl: papule
excl: insect bite S12; breast lump X19, Y16

S05 Lumps/swellings, generalized *R22.7, R23.8*

incl: papules/lumps/swellings in multiple sites
excl: swollen ankles/oedema K07

S06 Rash localized   *L53.9, R21*

incl: blotch, erythema, redness
excl: localized lump/swelling S05

S07 Rash generalized   *L53.9, R21*

incl: blotches/erythema/redness occurring in multiple sites
excl: other viral exanthem A76; generalized lumps/swellings skin S05

S08 Skin colour change   *L81.0 to L81.3, R23.0 to R23.2, R23.8*

incl: 'circles under eyes', cyanosis, flushing, freckles, pallor
excl: bruise S16; vitiligo S99

S09 Infected finger/toe   *L03.0*

incl: paronychia
excl: post-traumatic infection finger/toe S11; tinea S74; monilia/candida S75

S10 Boil/carbuncle   *L02*

incl: abscess, furuncle
excl: lymphadenitis B70; perianal boil D95; external auditory meatus H70; boil of
          nose R73; infected finger/toe, S09; wound infection S11; erysipelas S76;
          pilonidal abscess S85; hydradenitis S92; boil female external genitalia X99;
          boil male external genitalia Y99

S11 Skin infection, post-traumatic   *T79.3*

incl: infected post-traumatic wound/bite
excl: surgical wound infection A87; erysipelas pyoderma S76; impetigo S84

S12 Insect bite/sting

S00.0, S00.2 to S00.9, S10.1 to S10.9, S20.1, S20.3 to S20.8, S30.7 to S30.9,
S40.7, S40.8, S50.7, S50.8, S60.7, S60.8, S70.7, S70.8, S80.7, S80.8,
S90.7, S90.8, T09.0, T11.0, T13.0, T14.0

excl: toxic effects non-medical substance A86; infected bite S11; scabies S72;
          pediculosis S73

S13 Animal/human bite   *T14.1*

excl: toxic effects non-medical substance A86; infected bite S11

S14 Burn/scald   *T20 to T25, T30 to T32*

incl: burn/scald of all degrees; external chemical burn
excl: sunburn S80

S15 Foreign body in skin

S00.0, S00.2 to S00.9, S10.1 to S10.9, S20.1, S20.3 to S20.8, S30.7 to S30.9, S40.7, S40.8, S50.7, S50.8, S60.7, S60.8, S70.7, S70.8, S80.7, S80.8, S90.7, S90.8, T09.0, T11.0, T13.0, T14.0, T14.1

incl: foreign body under nail

S16 Bruise/contusion

S00.0, S00.8, S00.9, S10.0, S10.8, S10.9, S20.0, S20.2, S30.0, S30.1, S40.0, S50.0, S50.1, S60.0 to S60.2, S70.0, S70.1, S80.0, S80.1, S90.0 to S90.3, T09.0, T11.0, T13.0, T14.0

incl: ecchymosis, haematoma
excl: bruise/contusion with broken skin S17
criteria: bruise/contusion with intact skin surface

S17 Abrasion/scratch/blister

S00.0, S00.7 to S00.9, S10.1 to S10.9, S20.1, S20.3 to S20.8, S30.7 to S30.9, S40.7, S40.8, S50.7, S50.8, S60.7, S60.8, S70.7, S70.8, S80.7, S80.8, S90.7, S90.8, T09.0, T11.0, T13.0, T14.0

incl: bruise with broken skin, graze

S18 Laceration/cut

S01.0, S01.2, S01.4, S01.7 to S01.9, S11, S21, S31.0, S31.1, S31.8, S41, S51, S61, S71, S81, S91, T09.1, T11.1, T13.1, T14.1

incl: laceration/cut of skin/subcutaneous tissues
excl: bite S13; bruise with broken skin S17

S19 Skin injury, other

S00.0, S00.7 to S00.9, S10.1 to S10.9, S20.1, S20.3 to S20.8, S30.7 to S30.9, S40.7 to S40.9, S50.7 to S50.9, S60.7 to S60.9, S70.7 to S70.9, S80.7 to S80.9, S90.7 to S90.9, T09.0, T11.0, T13.0, T14.0, T14.1

incl: avulsion nail, needle stick, puncture
excl: bite S13

S20 Corn/callosity   *L84*

excl: hyperkeratosis S80

S21 Skin texture symptom/complaint   *R23.4*

incl: dry skin, peeling, scaling, wrinkles
excl: sweating problem A09; scalp symptom/complaint S24; ichthyosis S83; sweat gland disease S92; vulval symptom/complaint X16

S22 Nail symptom/complaint   *L60.1, L60.4, L60.5, L60.9, L62, R68.3*

incl: clubbing
excl: paronychia S09; ingrowing nail S94

S23 Hair loss/baldness   *L63 to L66*

incl: alopecia

S24 Hair/scalp symptom/complaint, other   *L67, L68*

incl: dry scalp, hirsutism
excl: tricotillomania P29; folliculitis S10; hair loss/baldness S23; dandruff S86

S26 Fear of cancer of skin   *Z71.1*

excl: if the patient has the disease, code the disease
criteria: concern about/fear of cancer of skin in a patient without the disease/until the diagnosis is proven

S27 Fear of skin disease, other   *Z71.1*

excl: fear of cancer of skin S26; if the patient has the disease, code the disease
criteria: concern about/fear of having other skin disease in a patient without the disease/until the diagnosis is proven

S28 Limited function/disability (S)   *Z73.6*

criteria: limitation of function/disability due to a skin problem
Note: The COOP/WONCA Charts are suitable for documenting the patient's functional status (see Chapter 8).

S29 Skin symptom/complaint, other   *R23.3, R23.8*

incl: cellulite, petechiae, problems with umbilicus, sore(s)
excl: scar S99

Component 7—Diagnosis/diseases

S70 Herpes zoster   *B02*

incl: post-herpetic neuralgia, shingles, herpes zoster ophthalmicus
criteria: grouped vesicular eruptions, unilateral distribution, over area of a single dermatome
consider: skin pain S01; localized rash S06

S71 Herpes simplex   *B00.0, B00.1, B00.2, B00.8, B00.9*

incl: cold sore, fever blister
excl: herpes simplex of eye without corneal ulcer F73; genital herpes X90, Y72
criteria: vesicles with erythematous base in localized area(s); plus past history of
             similar lesions, or virological or serological evidence
consider: localized rash S06

S72 Scabies/other acariasis   *B86, B88.0, B88.2*

criteria: intensely pruritic skin lesions plus arrays of burrows on sides of palms, fingers,
             penis, or skin folds; or demonstration of parasites or ova in lesions
consider: pruritus S02

S73 Pediculosis/skin infestation, other
B85, B87, B88.1, B88.3, B88.8, B88.9

incl: fleas, lice, mites, ticks
excl: infected insect bites S11; insect bites S12
criteria: demonstration of nits on hair shafts or insects on skin/clothes
consider: pruritus S02; localized rash S06

S74 Dermatophytosis   *B35, B36*

incl: fungal skin infection, onychomycosis, pityriasis versicolor, ringworm, tinea
excl: monilia/candida S75
criteria: pruritic scaly lesions with central clearing and small vesicles at border; or
             demonstration of fungus

S75 Moniliasis/candidiasis skin   *B37.2*

incl: monilial intertrigo, thrush involving nails/perianal region/skin
excl: oral thrush D83; genital candidiasis X72, Y75

S76 Skin infection, other
A46, A66, A67, L03.1 to L03.3, L03.8, L03.9, L08, L98.0

incl: cellulitis, erysipelas, pyoderma, strep skin infection
excl: boil/carbuncle S10; other localized skin infection S11; impetigo S84;
             molluscum contagiosum S95; acne S96

S77 Malignant neoplasm of skin   *C43, C44, C46.0*

incl: basal cell carcinoma, malignant melanoma, rodent ulcer, squamous cell
             carcinoma of skin
excl: premalignant lesion of skin S79   *(cont.)*

criteria: characteristic histological appearance
consider: other malignant neoplasm (when primary site is uncertain) A79; neoplasm of
              skin unspecified as benign or malignant/when histology is not available S79

S78 Lipoma   *D17*

S79 Neoplasm skin, benign/unspecified   *D03, D04, D23, D48.5*

incl: benign skin neoplasm, skin neoplasm not specified as benign or malignant/
          when histology is not available, dermoid cyst, premalignant lesion
excl: residual haemorrhoidal skin tag K96; solar keratosis S80; haemangioma
          S81; mole/pigmented naevus S82; keloid, hyperkeratosis, seborrhoeic/senile
          warts S99

S80 Solar keratosis/sunburn   *L55 to L59*

incl: photosensitivity, radiation skin damage, senile keratosis, solar hyperkerato-
          sis, polymorphous light eruption
excl: skin damage due to human-made radiation A87, A88

S81 Haemangioma/lymphangioma   *D18*

incl: angiomatous birthmark, portwine stain
criteria: vascular or lymphatic tumour, elevated above skin and emptying on pressure
consider: localized swelling S04

S82 Naevus/mole   *D22*

S83 Congenital skin anomaly, other   *Q80 to Q82, Q84*

incl: birthmark, ichthyosis
excl: haemangioma/lymphangioma S81

S84 Impetigo   *L00, L01*

incl: impetigo secondary to other dermatosis
criteria: spreading skin lesion consisting of macules, vesicles, pustules, or crust with
             underlying raw area
consider: other localized skin infection S11

S85 Pilonidal cyst/fistula   *L05*

incl: pilonidal abscess
excl: dermoid cyst S79

S86 Dermatitis, seborrhoeic   *L21*

incl: cradle cap, dandruff   *(cont.)*

excl: seborrhoeic warts S99
criteria: greasy, scaly lesions with underlying erythema on one or more areas of
             scalp, face, sternum, interscapular areas, around umbilicus and in body
             folds, not attributable to other skin disease
consider: localized rash S06; generalized rash S07

S87 Dermatitis, atopic eczema   *L20*

incl: flexural dermatitis, infantile eczema
excl: dermatitis/atopic eczema affecting external auditory meatus only H70;
             allergic dermatitis S88; diaper rash S89
criteria: pruritic exudative lesions with/without lichenification over face and neck,
             wrists and hands, chest, back of knees, and front of elbow
consider: pruritus S02; localized rash S06; generalized rash S07

S88 Dermatitis, contact/allergic
L23 to L25, L27.2, L27.8, L27.9, L30.0, L30.3, L30.4, L30.8, L30.9

incl: allergic dermatitis, chemical dermatitis, dermatitis NOS, eczema NOS,
             intertrigo, plant sting, skin allergy
excl: allergy/allergic reaction unspecified A92; contact/other dermatitis
             of eyelid F72; contact/other dermatitis of external auditory meatus H70;
             atopic eczema S87; diaper rash S89; urticaria S98; dermatitis artefacta/
             neurodermatitis S99
criteria: pruritic erythematous lesions related to exposure to chemical substance
consider: pruritus S02; localized rash S06; generalized rash S07

S89 Diaper rash   *L22*

criteria: dermatitis, primarily of the diaper area and sparing creases

S90 Pityriasis rosea   *L42*

criteria: oval, scaly eruptions along skin tension lines of trunk, with a history of
             a solitary lesion preceeding presenting rash
consider: localized rash S06; generalized rash S07

S91 Psoriasis   *L40*

criteria: plaques with silvery scales on knees, elbows, or scalp and/or stippled/pitted nails
Note: Double code psoriatic arthritis L99.

S92 Sweat gland disease   *L30.1, L73.2, L74, L75*

incl: dyshidrosis, heat rash, hydradenitis, miliaria, pompholyx, prickly heat,
             sweat rash
excl: hyperhidrosis A09

S93 Sebaceous cyst   *L72.1*

incl: wen

S94 Ingrowing nail   *L60.0*

excl: paronychia S09

S95 Molluscum contagiosum   *B08.1*

S96 Acne   *L70*

incl: blackheads, comedones, pimples
excl: acne due to medication A85

S97 Chronic ulcer skin   *I83.0, I83.2, L89, L97, L98.4*

incl: bedsore, decubitus ulcer, pressure sore, varicose ulcer
excl: gangrene K92

S98 Urticaria   *L50*

incl: hives, weals
excl: drug allergy A85; angioedema/allergic oedema A92

S99 Skin disease, other

L10 to L14, L26, L28, L30.2, L30.5, L41, L43 to L45, L51, L52, L53.0 to L53.3, L53.8, L54, L60.2, L60.3, L60.8, L71, L72.0, L72.2, L72.8, L72.9, L73.0, L73.1, L73.8, L73.9, L80, L81.4 to L81.9, L82, L83, L85 to L88, L90 to L95, L98.1 to L98.3, L98.5 to L98.9, L99

incl: dermatitis artefacta, discoid lupus erythematosus, erythema multiforme, erythema nodosum, folliculitis, granuloma, granuloma annulare, hyper-keratosis NOS, keloid, keratoacanthoma, lichen planus, neurodermatitis, onychogryphosis, rosacea, pigmentation, rhinophyma, scar, seborrhoeic or senile warts, striae atrophicae, vitiligo

T Endocrine, metabolic and nutritional

Component—Symptoms and complaints

T01 Excessive thirst   *R63.1*

incl: polydipsia

T02 Excessive appetite   *R63.2*

incl: overeating, polyphagia
excl: bulimia P86

T03 Loss of appetite   *R63.0*

incl: anorexia
excl: anorexia nervosa P86

T04 Feeding problem of infant/child   *R63.3*

incl: problem of what and how to eat/feed infant/child
excl: food allergy A92; food intolerance D99; feeding problem/eating disorders
            with psychological cause P11

T05 Feeding problem of adult   *R63.3*

incl: problem of what and how to eat/feed adult
excl: food allergy A92; dysphagia D21; food intolerance D99; psychological eating
            disorders/food refusal P29; anorexia/bulimia nervosa P86; loss of appetite T03

T07 Weight gain   *R63.5*

excl: obesity T82; overweight T83

T08 Weight loss   *R63.4, R64*

incl: cachexia
excl: anorexia nervosa P86

T10 Growth delay   *E34.3, R62.8, R62.9*

incl: failure to thrive, physiological delay growth
excl: delayed milestones P22; learning disorder P24; mental retardation P85;
            delayed puberty T99

T11 Dehydration   *E86*

incl: water depletion
excl: salt depletion/electrolyte disturbance T99

T26 Fear of cancer of endocrine system   *Z71.1*

excl: if the patient has the disease, code the disease
criteria: concern about/fear of cancer of endocrine system in a patient without the
            disease/until the diagnosis is proven

T27 Fear of endocrine/metabolic disease, other   *Z71.1*

incl: fear of diabetes
excl: fear of cancer of endocrine system T26; if the patient has the disease, code
             the disease
criteria: concern about/fear of other endocrine/metabolic/nutritional disease in a
             patient without the disease/until the diagnosis is proven

T28 Limited function/disability (T)   *Z73.6*

criteria: limited function/disability due to a problem of the endocrine/metabolic/
             nutritional system
Note: The COOP/WONCA Charts are suitable for documenting the patient's functional
status (see Chapter 8).

T29 Endocrine/metabolic/nutritional symptom/complaint, other   *R63.8*

incl: specific food craving, underweight
excl: hyperglycaemia A91; fluid retention K07

Component 7—Diagnosis/diseases

T70 Endocrine infection   *E06.0*

excl: thyroiditis T99

T71 Malignant neoplasm thyroid   *C73*

criteria: characteristic histological appearance
consider: other/unspecified endocrine neoplasm T73; goitre T81

T72 Benign neoplasm thyroid   *D34*

excl: other/unspecified endocrine neoplasm T73; goitre T81

T73 Neoplasm endocrine, other/unspecified   *C74, C75, D09.3, D35, D44*

T78 Thyroglossal duct/cyst   *Q89.2*
excl: goitre T81

T80 Congenital anomaly endocrine/metabolic   *E00, Q89.1, Q89.2*

incl: cretinism, dwarfism
excl: thyroglossal duct (cyst) T78

T81 Goitre   *E04*

incl: non-toxic goitre, thyroid nodule
excl: neoplasm of thyroid gland T71–T73; thyroglossal cyst T78; toxic goitre
             T85; hypothyroidism T86

T82 Obesity   *E66*

excl: overweight T83
criteria: a body mass index greater than 30

T83 Overweight   *E66*

excl: obesity T82
criteria: a body mass index greater than 25 but less than 30

T85 Hyperthyroidism/thyrotoxicosis   *E05*

incl: Graves' disease, toxic goitre
excl: non-toxic goitre T81
criteria: laboratory evidence of excessive thyroid hormone; or thyroid nodule or
             goitre plus tremor, weight loss, and rapid pulse (over 100/min at rest) or eye
             signs (exophthalmos, lid lag, or ophthamoplegia)

T86 Hypothyroidism/myxoedema   *E01 to E03*

excl: cretinism T80
criteria: laboratory evidence of diminished thyroid hormone activity and excessive
             thyroid stimulating hormone; or four or more of the following: weakness/
             tiredness; mental changes: apathy, poor memory, slowing; voice changes:
             coarser, deeper slower speech; undue sensitivity to cold; constipation; coarse
             puffy facial features; cool dry, sallow skin, decreased sweating; peripheral
             oedema
consider: other complaint of metabolism T29

T87 Hypoglycaemia   *E15, E16.0 to E16.3, E16.9*

incl: hyperinsulism, insulin coma
criteria: hypoglycaemia demonstrated by biochemical testing, or characteristic
             symptoms in a diabetic patient relieved by ingestion or injection of sugar

T89 Diabetes, insulin dependent   *E10*

incl: juvenile-onset diabetes, type 1 diabetes
excl: drug-induced hyperglycaemia A85; hyperglycaemia as isolated finding A91;
             non-insulin dependent diabetes T90; gestational diabetes W85

(cont.)

criteria: patient requiring regular ongoing treatment with insulin after diagnosis confirmed by one of the following:

(a) the classic symptoms of diabetes, such as polyuria, polydipsia, and rapid weight loss, together with unequivocal elevation of plasma glucose

(b) fasting blood glucose levels of 8 mmol/L (140 mg/dL) or more on two or more occasions

(c) random blood glucose levels of 11 mmol/L (200 mg/dL) or more on two or more occasions

(d) an oral glucose tolerance test (75 g glucose) with one value of plasma glucose concentration at between 1 and 2 h of 11 mmol/L (200 mg/dL) or more, and plasma glucose level at 2 h of 11 mol/L (200 mg/dL) or more; these WHO criteria may change over time; also, criteria differences may exist between national health care systems

Note: (1) Double code complications such as retinopathy F83, nephropathy U88; (2) in pregnancy, double code with W84.

T90 Diabetes, non-insulin dependent   *E11 to E14*

 incl: diabetes NOS, late-onset diabetes, type 2 diabetes
excl: drug-induced hyperglycaemia A85; hyperglycaemia as isolated finding A91; insulin-dependent diabetes T89; gestational diabetes W85
criteria: patient not requiring regular ongoing treatment with insulin after diagnosis confirmed by one of the following:

(a) the classical symptoms of diabetes, such as polyuria, polydipsia, and rapid weight loss, together with unequivocal increase in plasma glucose concentration

(b) fasting blood glucose level of 8 mmol/L (140 mg/dL) or more on two or more occasions

(c) random blood glucose level of 11 mmol/L (200 mg/dL) or more on two or more occasions

(d) an oral glucose tolerance test (75 g glucose) one value of plasma glucose concentration at between 1 and 2 h of 11 mmol/L (200 mg/dL) or more and plasma glucose level at 2 h of 11 mol/L (200 mg/dL) or more; these WHO criteria may change over time; also, criteria differences may exist between national health care systems

Note: (1) Double code complications such as retinopathy F83, nephropathy U88; (2) in pregnancy, double code with W84.

T91 Vitamin/nutritional deficiency
E40 to E46, E50, E51.1, E51.8, E51.9, E52 to E56,
E58 to E61, E63, E64

incl: beri-beri, dietary mineral deficiency, iron deficiency without anaemia, malnutrition, marasmus, scurvy   *(cont.)*

excl:　　iron deficiency anaemia B80; pernicious anaemia B81; malabsorption syndrome/sprue D99

T92 Gout　　　　　　　　　　　　　　　　　　　　　　　*M10*

excl:　　drug-induced gout A85; raised uric acid A91; pseudo-gout/other crystal arthropathy T99

T93 Lipid disorder　　　　　　　　　　　　　　　　　　*E78*

incl:　　abnormality of lipoprotein level, hyperlipidaemia, raised level of cholesterol/triglycerides, xanthoma

T99 Endocrine/metabolic/nutritional disease, other
E06.1 to E06.5, E06.9, E07, E16.8, E20 to E32, E34.0 to E34.2, E34.4 to E34.9, E35, E65, E67, E68, E70 to E77, E79, E80, E83 to E85, E87, E88, E90, M11, M83

incl:　　acromegaly, adrenal/ovarian/pituitary/parathyroid/testicular/other endocrine dysfunction, amyloidosis, crystal arthropathy, Cushing's syndrome, cystic fibrosis, diabetes insipidus, Gilbert's syndrome, hyperaldosteronism, osteomalacia, porphyria, precocious/delayed puberty, pseudo-gout, renal glycosuria, thyroiditis

excl:　　food allergy A92; food intolerance D99; osteoporosis L95

U Urinary system

Component 1—Symptoms and complaints

U01 Dysuria/painful urination　　　　　　　　　　　　*R30*

incl:　　burning urination
excl:　　frequent/urgent urination U02; urethritis U72

U02 Urinary frequency/urgency　　　　　　　　　　　　*R35*

incl:　　nocturia, polyuria

U04 Incontinence urine　　　　　　　　　　　*N39.3, N39.4, R32*

incl:　　enuresis of organic origin, involuntary urination, stress incontinence
excl:　　urine incontinence of psychogenic origin P12

U05 Urination problems, other　　　　　　　　　　　*R34, R39.1*

incl:　　anuria, dribbling urine, oliguria
excl:　　urinary retention U08

U06 Haematuria   *N02, R31*

incl: blood in urine
criteria: blood in urine proven by macroscopic/microscopic/chemical test

U07 Urine symptom/complaint, other   *R39.8*

incl: bad odour of urine, dark urine
excl: abnormal urine test U98

U08 Urinary retention   *R33*

U13 Bladder symptom/complaint, other   *R39.0, R39.8*

incl: bladder pain, irritable bladder

U14 Kidney symptom/complaint   *N23*

incl: kidney pain, kidney trouble, renal colic
excl: loin/flank pain L05

U26 Fear of cancer of urinary system   *Z71.1*

excl: if the patient has the disease, code the disease
criteria: concern about/fear of urinary cancer in a patient without the disease/until
            the diagnosis is proven

U27 Fear of urinary disease, other   *Z71.1*

excl: fear of cancer of urinary system U26; if the patient has the disease, code the
            disease
criteria: concern about/fear of other urinary disease in a patient without the disease/
            until the diagnosis is proven

U28 Limited function/disability (U)   *Z73.6, Z99.2*

incl: renal transplant, slow stream
excl: urinary incontinence U04
criteria: limitation of function/disability due to a urinary problem
Note: The COOP/WONCA Charts are suitable for documenting the patient's functional
status (see Chapter 8).

U29 Urinary symptom/complaint, other   *R39.8*

excl: irritable bladder/bladder pain U13; kidney symptom/complaint U14

Component 7—Diagnosis/diseases

U70 Pyelonephritis/pyelitis   *N10 to N12, N15.1, N15.9*

incl: infection of kidney, renal/perinephric abscess
criteria: two or more of the following: flank pain, renal tenderness, investigation
            evidence of chronic renal damage; plus clinical or laboratory evidence of
            urinary tract infection
consider: cystitis/other urinary infection U71

U71 Cystitis/urinary infection, other   *N30, N39.0*

incl: acute/chronic cystitis (non-venereal), asymptomatic bacteriuria, lower urinary
            tract infection, urinary tract infection NOS
excl: pyelonephritis U70; urethritis U72; vaginitis X84; balanitis Y75
Note: In pregnancy, also code W84.

U72 Urethritis   *A56.0, A56.2, A59.0, B37.4, N34*

incl: chlamydial urethritis in man, non-specific urethritis, urethral syndrome,
            meatitis
excl: gonococcal urethritis female X71; urethritis chlamydial female X92; urethritis
            trichomonal female X73; gonococcal urethritis male Y71
criteria: urethral discharge with frequency, burning, pain or urgency on urination
            without bacteruria by microscopy or culture; or inflammation of external
            urinary meatus
consider: painful urination U01; frequent/urgent urination U02; irritable bladder U13;
            urethral discharge X29, Y03

U75 Malignant neoplasm kidney   *C64, C65*

criteria: characteristic histological appearance
consider: neoplasm urinary tract NOS U79

U76 Malignant neoplasm bladder   *C67*

criteria: characteristic histological appearance
consider: neoplasm urinary tract NOS U79

U77 Malignant neoplasm urinary, other   *C66, C68*

incl: malignant neoplasm ureter, malignant neoplasm urethra
excl: malignant neoplasm prostate Y77
criteria: characteristic histological appearance
consider: neoplasm urinary tract NOS U79

U78 Benign neoplasm urinary tract   *D30*

incl: bladder papilloma, polyp of urinary tract
excl: prostatic hypertrophy Y85
criteria: characteristic histological appearance
consider: neoplasm urinary tract NOS U79

U79 Neoplasm urinary tract, unspecified   *D09.0, D09.1, D41*

incl: neoplasm of bladder/kidney/ureter/urethra not specified as benign or malignant/
             when histology is not available
excl: malignant neoplasm kidney U75; malignant neoplasm bladder U76; other
             malignant urinary neoplasm U77; benign urinary neoplasm U78

U80 Injury urinary tract   *S37.0 to S37.3, T19.0, T19.1, T28.3, T28.8*

incl: contusion kidney, foreign body in urinary tract

U85 Congenital anomaly urinary tract   *Q60 to Q64*

incl: duplex kidney/ureter, congenital polycystic kidney

U88 Glomerulonephritis/nephrosis
                               N00, N01, N03 to N05, N07, N08, N14, N15.0, N15.8, N16

incl: acute glomerulonephritis, analgesic nephropathy, chronic glomerulonephritis,
             nephritis, nephropathy, nephrosclerosis, nephrotic syndrome
excl: renal failure U99
criteria: three or more of the following: haematuria, proteinuria, renal salt and water
             retention, decreased renal function, persistent urinary sediment abnormalities;
             or renal biopsy evidence
consider: abnormal urine test result U98; kidney symptom/complaint U14

U90 Orthostatic albuminuria/proteinuria   *N39.2*

incl: postural proteinuria
criteria: albuminuria following ambulation, no albuminuria following overnight
             recumbency and no evidence of renal disease
consider: proteinuria NOS U98

U95 Urinary calculus   *N20 to N22*

incl: calculus/stone in bladder/kidney/ureter, urolithiasis
criteria: colicky pain and either haematuria or history of urinary stone in the past; or
             passage of calculus; or imaging evidence of calculus
consider: blood in urine U06; renal colic U14; other urinary symptom U29; abnormal
             urine test U98

U98 Abnormal urine test NOS   *N39.1, R80 to R82*

incl: glycosuria, proteinuria, pus in urine, pyuria
excl: haematuria/blood in urine U06; orthostatic albuminuria/proteinuria U90

U99 Urinary disease, other
                 N06, N13, N17 to N19, N25 to N29, N31 to N33, N35 to N37, N39.8,
                                N39.9, R39.2, T19.8, T19.9, Z90.5, Z90.6

incl: bladder diverticulum, hydronephrosis, hypertrophic kidney, obstruction
            bladder neck, renal failure, urethral caruncle, urethral stricture, ureteric
            reflux, uraemia

W Pregnancy, childbearing, family planning

Component 1—Symptoms and complaints

W01 Question of pregnancy   *Z32.0*

incl: delayed menstruation, symptoms suggestive of pregnancy
excl: fear of pregnancy W02; pregnancy confirmed W78, W79

W02 Fear of pregnancy   *Z71.1*

incl: concern about possibility of unwanted pregnancy
excl: concern/fear if unwanted pregnancy confirmed W79

W03 Antepartum bleeding   *O20, O46*

W05 Pregnancy vomiting/nausea   *O21*

incl: hyperemesis, morning sickness in confirmed pregnancy

W10 Contraception, post-coital   *Z30.3*

incl: morning after pill

W11 Contraception, oral   *Z30.4*

incl: family planning in woman using oral hormonal therapy

W12 Contraception, intrauterine   *Z30.1, Z30.5*

incl: family planning using IUD

W13 Sterilization female   *Z30.2*

incl: family planning involving female sterilization

W14 Contraception female, other   *Z30.0, Z30.8, Z30.9*

incl: contraception NOS, family planning NOS
excl: genetic counselling A98; oral contraception W11; IUD W12; family planning
            by female sterilization W13

W15 Infertility/subfertility female   *N97, Z31.0 to Z31.4, Z31.6 to Z31.9*

incl: sterility, primary and secondary
criteria: failure to conceive after 2 years of trying
consider: other symptom/complaint about pregnancy W29

W17 Post-partum bleeding   *O72*

criteria: heavy bleeding at or within 6 weeks of parturition
consider: other post-partum complaints W18

W18 Post-partum symptom/complaint, other   *O90.9*

excl: puerperal depression P76; post-partum bleeding W17; lactation complaints
              W19; complications of puerperium W96
criteria: complaints related to and within 6 weeks of parturition

W19 Breast/lactation symptom/complaint   *O92.5 to O92.7*

incl: galactorrhoea, suppression of lactation, weaning
excl: puerperal mastitis W94; cracked nipples W95

W21 Concern about body image related to pregnancy   *R46.8*

W27 Fear of complications of pregnancy   *Z71.1*

incl: fear of congenital anomaly in baby
excl: if the patient has the complication, code the complication
criteria: concern about/fear of complications in a patient without them/until they are
              proven

W28 Limited function/disability (W)   *Z73.6*

incl: pelvic instability
criteria: limitation of function/disability due to or related to pregnancy
Note: The COOP/WONCA Charts are suitable for documenting the patient's functional
status (see Chapter 8).

W29 Pregnancy symptom/complaint, other   *O26*

incl: family planning symptom/complaint, other

Component 7—Diagnoses

W70 Puerperal infection/sepsis   *O85, O86.1, O86.3*

excl: obstetric tetanus N72
criteria: infection of birth canal or reproductive organs within 6 weeks of parturition

W71 Other infection complicating pregnancy/puerperium
O23, O41.1, O75.2, O75.3, O86.2, O86.4, O86.8, O98

excl: puerperal infection W70; puerperal mastitis W94

W72 Malignant neoplasm related to pregnancy   *C58*

incl: chorioepithelioma, choriocarcinoma

W73 Benign/unspecified neoplasm related to pregnancy   *O01*

incl: benign neoplasm related to pregnancy, neoplasm related to pregnancy
           not specified as benign or malignant/when histology is not available, hydati-
           diform mole

W75 Injury complicating pregnancy   *T14.9*

incl: results of injury interfering with pregnancy
excl: new injury caused by childbirth W92, W93

W76 Congenital anomaly complicating pregnancy   *O99.8*

incl: maternal anomaly that could affect pregnancy/childbirth

W78 Pregnancy   *Z32.1, Z33, Z34, Z36*

incl: pregnancy confirmed
excl: unwanted pregnancy W79; ectopic pregnancy W80; high risk pregnancy W84

W79 Unwanted pregnancy   *Z32.1, Z64.0*

W80 Ectopic pregnancy   *O00*

criteria: confirmation by ultrasonography, laparoscopy, culdoscopy or surgery
consider: antepartum bleeding W03, other symptom/complaint in pregnancy W29

W81 Toxaemia of pregnancy   *O10 to O16*

incl: eclampsia, hypertension, oedema and proteinuria in pregnancy, pre-eclampsia
consider: other symptom/complaint in pregnancy W29

W82 Abortion, spontaneous   *O02, O03, O05, O06*

incl: abortion threatened/complete/incomplete/missed/habitual, miscarriage
excl: ante-partum bleeding W03; induced abortion W83; premature contractions
           after the 28th week of pregnancy W92; fetal death/stillbirth after the 28th
           week of pregnancy W93

W83 Abortion, induced   *O04, Z30.3*

incl: termination of pregnancy, all complications

W84 Pregnancy high risk
           O24.0 to O24.3, O24.9, O25, O30 to O36, O40, O43, O44, O99.0 to O99.7, Z35

incl: aged primipara, anaemia of pregnancy, diabetes/other pre-existing chronic
           disease affecting pregnancy, disproportion, hydramnios, malpresentation,
           multiple pregnancy, placenta praevia, previous caesarian section, premature
           labour, small fetus for age
excl: infections complicating pregnancy W71; ectopic pregnancy W80; toxaemia
           of pregnancy W81; gestational diabetes W85

W85 Gestational diabetes   *O24.4*

incl: diabetes manifested during pregnancy
excl: pre-existing diabetes T89, T90
criteria: fasting plasma glucose level over 5.5 mmol/L and/or plasma glucose level
           greater than 8.0 mmol/L 2 h after a 75-g oral glucose tolerance test
consider: hyperglycaemia A91

W90 Uncomplicated labour/delivery, livebirth   *O80, Z37.0, Z37.9, Z38, Z39*

W91 Uncomplicated labour/delivery, stillbirth   *Z37.1, Z37.9*

W92 Complicated labour/delivery, livebirth
           O42, O45, O60 to O71, O73, O75.0, O75.1, O75.4 to O75.9, O81 to O84, Z37.2,
           Z37.5, Z37.9, Z38, Z39

incl: livebirth after complicated delivery: assisted extraction, breech delivery,
           caesarian section, dystocia, induction of labour, injuries caused by child-
           birth, placenta praevia in delivery, version
excl: post-partum haemorrhage W17; eclampsia W81

W93 Complicated labour/delivery, stillbirth
           O42, O45, O60 to O71, O73, O75.0, O75.1, O75.4 to O75.9, O81 to O84,
           Z37.1, Z37.3, Z37.4, Z37.6, Z37.7, Z37.9

incl: stillbirth after complicated delivery: assisted extraction, breech delivery,
           caesarian section, dystocia, induction of labour, injuries caused by child-
           birth, placenta praevia in delivery, version
excl: post-partum haemorrhage W17; eclampsia W81

W94 Puerperal mastitis   *O91*

incl: breast abscess
criteria: pain, inflammation of breast within 6 weeks of parturition or while lactating
consider: disorders of lactation W19

W95 Breast disorder in pregnancy/puerperium, other   *O92.0 to O92.4*

incl: breast disorder in puerperium, cracked nipple
excl: disorders of lactation W19; mastitis W94; breast problem not related to
         pregnancy/lactation X21

W96 Complications of puerperium, other   *O87, O90.4, O90.8, O90.9*

excl: puerperal depression P76; puerperal psychosis P98; puerperal infection
         W70; toxaemia of pregnancy W81; breast disorder in pregnancy W95

W99 Disorder of pregnancy/delivery, other
O07, O08, O22, O26, O28, O41.0, O41.8, O41.9, O47, O48,
O88, O90.5, O95 to O97

excl: pseudocyesis P75

X Female genital system (including breast)

Component 1—Symptoms and complaints

X01 Genital pain female   *N94.8*

incl: pelvic pain, vulval pain
excl: menstrual pain X02; dyspareunia female X04; breast pain female X18

X02 Menstrual pain   *N94.4 to N94.6*

incl: dysmenorrhoea

X03 Intermenstrual pain   *N94.0*

incl: Mittelschmerz, ovulation pain

X04 Painful intercourse female   *N94.1, N94.2*

incl: female dyspareunia, vaginismus NOS
excl: psychogenic sexual problems P07, P08

X05 Menstruation absent/scanty   *N91*

incl: amenorrhoea, delayed/late menses, oligomenorrhoea
excl: question of pregnancy W01; fear of pregnancy W02

X06 Menstruation excessive   *N92.0, N92.2, N92.4*

incl: menorrhagia, pubertal bleeding

X07 Menstruation irregular/frequent   *N92.0, N92.1, N92.5, N92.6*

incl: polymenorrhoea
excl: menorrhagia/pubertal bleeding X06

X08 Intermenstrual bleeding   *N92.3, N93.8, N93.9*

incl: breakthrough bleeding, dysfunctional uterine bleeding, metrorrhagia, ovula-
              tion bleeding, spotting
excl: post-menopausal bleeding X12; post-coital bleeding X13

X09 Premenstrual symptom/complaint   *N94.8, N94.9*

excl: premenstrual tension syndrome X89

X10 Postponement of menstruation   *Z30.9*

criteria: postponement of the expected regular menstruation by hormonal treatment

X11 Menopausal symptom/complaint   *N95.1 to N95.3, N95.8, N95.9*

incl: atrophic vaginitis, menopause syndrome, symptom/complaint related to
              menopause, senile vaginitis
excl: post-menopausal bleeding X12

X12 Post-menopausal bleeding   *N95.0*

criteria: vaginal bleeding following either at least 6 months' amenorrhoea or demon-
              stration of menopause by appropriate laboratory test
consider: irregular menstruation X07

X13 Post-coital bleeding   *N93.0*

incl: contact bleeding

X14 Vaginal discharge   *N89.8*

incl: fluor vaginalis, leukorrhoea
excl: vaginal bleeding X06, X07, X08; atrophic vaginitis X11; gonorrhoea female
              X71; urogenital candidiasis female X72; urogenital trichomoniasis female
              X73; chlamydia genital female X92

X15 Vaginal symptom/complaint, other   *N89.8, N89.9*

incl: vaginal dryness
excl: female genital pain X01; organic vaginismus X04; atrophic vaginitis X11

X16 Vulval symptom/complaint   *L29.2, N90.9*

incl: vulval pruritus, vulval dryness
excl: vulval pain X01; abscess vulva X99

X17 Pelvis symptom/complaint female   *N94.8, N94.9*

excl: genital pain female X01

X18 Breast pain female   *N64.4*

incl: mastodynia
excl: breast pain in pregnancy/lactation W19

X19 Breast lump/mass female   *N63*

incl: lumpy breasts

X20 Nipple symptom/complaint female   *N64.0, N64.5*

incl: nipple discharge, nipple fissure, nipple pain/pruritus, nipple retraction
excl: nipple symptom/complaint in pregnancy/lactation W19

X21 Breast symptom/complaint female, other

N61, N62, N64.3, N64.5, N64.8, N64.9

incl: mastitis (non-lactating), mastopathy, galactorrhoea
excl: mastitis (lactating) W94

X22 Concern about breast appearance female   *R46.8*

X23 Fear of sexually transmitted disease female   *Z71.1*

excl: fear of HIV/AIDS B25; if the patient has the disease, code the disease
criteria: concern about/fear of sexually transmitted disease in a patient without the
              disease/until the diagnosis is proven

X24 Fear of sexual dysfunction female   *Z71.1*

excl: sexual dysfunction P07, P08
criteria: concern about/fear of sexual dysfunction in a patient without sexual
              dysfunction

X25 Fear of genital cancer female   *Z71.1*

excl: if the patient has the disease, code the disease
criteria: concern about/fear of female genital cancer in a patient without the disease/
              until the diagnosis is proven

X26 Fear of breast cancer female   *Z71.1*

excl: if the patient has the disease, code the disease
criteria: concern about/fear of female breast cancer in a patient without the
              disease/until the diagnosis is proven

X27 Fear genital/breast disease female, other   *Z71.1*

excl: fear of female genital cancer X25; fear of female breast cancer X26; if the
              patient has the disease, code the disease
criteria: concern about/fear of other female genital/breast disease in a patient without
              the disease/until the diagnosis is proven

X28 Limited function/disability (X)   *Z73.6, Z90.7*

excl: sexual dysfunction P07, P08; painful intercourse female/vaginismus X04
criteria: limitation of function/disability due to a problem of the female genital
              system (including breast)
Note: The COOP/WONCA Charts are suitable for documenting the patient's functional
status (see Chapter 8).

X29 Genital symptom/complaint female, other   *N94.8, N94.9, R36*

incl: urethral discharge in female

Component 7—Diagnosis/diseases

X70 Syphilis female   *A50 to A53, A65, N74.2*

incl: syphilis any site
criteria: demonstration of *Treponema pallidum* on microscopy, or positive serological
              test for syphilis

X71 Gonorrhoea female   *A54, N74.3*

incl: gonorrhoea any site
criteria: purulent vaginal discharge in a patient after a contact with a proven case; or
              Gram-negative intracellular diplococci demonstrated in discharge; or culture
              of *Neisseria gonorrhoea*
consider: urethritis U72; urethral discharge female X29

X72 Genital candidiasis female   *B37.3, B37.4*

incl: monilial infection of vagina/cervix, thrush
criteria: inflamed urogenital mucosa or skin with characteristic white adherent
            exudate; or demonstration of candida
consider: vaginal discharge X14; vaginitis X84

X73 Genital trichomoniasis female   *A59.0*

criteria: characteristic foul-smelling discharge; or demonstration of trichomonads on
            microscopy
consider: vaginal discharge X14; vaginitis X84

X74 Pelvic inflammatory disease   *N70, N71, N73, N74.8*

incl: endometritis, oophoritis, salpingitis
excl: sexually transmitted diseases female X70–X73; chlamydia infection
            female X92
criteria: lower abdominal pain with marked tenderness of uterus or adnexa by palpa-
            tion, plus other evidence of inflammation
consider: pelvic congestion syndrome X99

X75 Malignant neoplasm cervix   *C53*

excl: carcinoma-in-situ cervix X81; cervical intraepithelial neoplasia (CIN) grade 3
            X81; abnormal cervix smear (CIN) grades 1 and 2 X86
criteria: characteristic histological appearance

X76 Malignant neoplasm breast female   *C50*

incl: intraductal carcinoma
excl: carcinoma-in-situ X81
criteria: characteristic histological appearance
consider: breast lump X19

X77 Malignant neoplasm genital female, other   *C51, C52, C54 to C57*

incl: malignancy of adnexae, ovaries, uterus, vagina, vulva
excl: carcinoma in-situ X81
criteria: characteristic histological appearance
consider: other/unspecified female genital neoplasm X81

X78 Fibromyoma uterus   *D25*

incl: fibroid uterus, fibromyoma of cervix, myoma
criteria: enlargement of the uterus not due to pregnancy or malignancy, with single or
            multiple firm tumours of the uterus

X79 Benign neoplasm breast female   *D24*

incl: fibroadenoma
excl: cystic disease of breast X88
criteria: characteristic histological appearance
consider: lump in female breast X19

X80 Benign neoplasm female, genital   *D26 to D28*

excl: polyp of cervix X85; physiological cyst of ovary X99

X81 Genital neoplasm female, other/unspecified
                                          D05, D06, D07.0 to D07.3, D39, D48.6

incl: carcinoma-in-situ, biopsy-proven cervical intraepithelial neoplasia (CIN)
             grade 3, female genital neoplasm not specified as benign or malignant/when
             histology is not available
excl: endometrial polyp X99

X82 Injury genital female
     S30.2, S31.4, S31.5, S37.4 to S37.6, S38.0, S38.2, S39.8, S39.9, T19.2, T19.3, T28.3, T28.8

incl: foreign body in vagina, female circumcision
excl: genital injury due to childbirth W92, W93

X83 Congenital anomaly genital female   *Q50 to Q52, Q56, Q83*

incl: hermaphroditism, imperforate hymen
excl: other genetic syndrome A90

X84 Vaginitis/vulvitis NOS   *N76, N77*

incl: vaginosis, gardnerella
excl: atrophic vaginitis X11; genital candidiasis female X72; genital trichomoniasis
             female X73

X85 Cervical disease NOS   *N72, N84.1, N86, N88*

incl: cervical erosion, cervical leukoplakia, cervicitis, mucous cervical polyp, old
             laceration of cervix
excl: abnormality of cervix in pregnancy/childbirth/puerperium W76; abnormal
             cervix smear X86

X86 Abnormal cervix smear   *N87, R87*

incl: cervical intraepithelial neoplasia (CIN) grades 1 and 2, cervical dysplasia
excl: cervical intraepithelial neoplasia (CIN) grade 3 X81

X87 Uterovaginal prolapse   *N81*

incl: cystocoele, procidentia, rectocoele
excl: stress incontinence U04

X88 Fibrocystic disease breast   *N60, N64.8, N64.9*

incl: chronic cystic disease of breast, cystic fibroadenosis of breast, dysplasia of
            breast, solitary cyst of breast

X89 Premenstrual tension syndrome   *N94.3*

criteria: cyclic occurrence in the menstrual cycle of two or more of the following:
              oedema; breast tenderness/swelling; headache; irritability; mood changes
consider: premenstrual symptom X09

X90 Genital herpes female   *A60*

incl: anogenital herpes simplex
criteria: small vesicles with characteristic appearance and location that evolve to
              painful ulcers and scabs

X91 Condylomata acuminata female   *A63.0*

incl: venereal warts, human papilloma virus infection
criteria: characteristic appearance of lesions, or characteristic histological appearance

X92 Chlamydia infection, genital female   *A56.0 to A56.4, A56.8, N74.4*

criteria: proven chlamydial infection

X99 Genital disease female, other
                A55, A57, A58, A63.8, N61, N64.1, N64.2, N64.8, N64.9, N75, N80, N82,
                N83, N84.0, N84.2, N84.3, N84.8, N84.9, N85, N89.0 to N89.7, N90.0 to
                N90.8, N94.8, N94.9, N96, N98, Z90.1, Z90.7

incl: Bartholin cyst/abscess, endometriosis, genital tract fistula female, pelvic
            congestion syndrome, physiological ovarian cyst
excl: sexually transmitted disease NOS A78

Y Male genital system

Component 1—Symptoms and complaints

Y01 Pain in penis   *N48.8*

excl: priapism/painful erection Y08

Y02 Pain in testis/scrotum   *R10.2, N50.8*

incl: pain perineum, pain pelvis

Y03 Urethral discharge male   *R36*

Y04 Penis symptom/complaint, other   *N48.8, N48.9*

incl: foreskin symptom/complaint
excl: pain in penis Y01; painful erection/priapism Y08

Y05 Scrotum/testis symptom/complaint, other   *L29.1, N50.8, N50.9*

incl: lump in testis
excl: pain in testis/scrotum Y02

Y06 Prostate symptom/complaint   *N42.8, N42.9*

incl: prostatism
excl: urinary frequency/urgency U02; urinary retention U08

Y07 Impotence NOS   *N48.4*

incl: impotence of organic origin
excl: reduced sexual desire P07; psychogenic impotence/reduced sexual fulfil-
            ment P08

Y08 Sexual function symptom/complaint male   *N48.3, N48.8*

incl: painful erection, priapism
excl: reduced sexual desire P07; psychogenic impotence/reduced sexual fulfil-
            ment P08; impotence of organic origin Y07

Y10 Infertility/subfertility male   *N46, Z31.0, Z31.4 to Z31.9*

criteria: failure of conception after 2 years of trying

Y13 Sterilization male   *Z30.2*

incl: family planning involving male sterilization

Y14 Family planning male, other   *Z30.0, Z30.8, Z30.9*

incl: contraception NOS, family planning NOS
excl: genetic counselling A98

Y16 Breast symptom/complaint male   *N62, N63, N64.5*

incl: gynaecomastia, lump breast
excl: disease of male breast Y99

Y24 Fear of sexual dysfunction male   *Z71.1*

excl: if the patient has sexual dysfunction, code the condition
criteria: concern about/fear of sexual dysfunction in a patient without the condition

Y25 Fear of sexually transmitted disease male   *Z71.1*

excl: fear of HIV/AIDS B25; in a patient with the disease, code the disease
criteria: concern about/fear of venereal disease in a patient without the disease/until
             the diagnosis is proven

Y26 Fear of genital cancer male   *Z71.1*

excl: in a patient with the disease, code the disease
criteria: concern about/fear of cancer in a patient without the disease/until the diag-
             nosis is proven

Y27 Fear of genital disease male, other   *Z71.1*

excl: fear of sexually transmitted disease Y25; fear of male genital cancer Y26; in
             a patient with the disease, code the disease
criteria: concern about/fear of other genital disease in a patient without the
             disease/until the diagnosis is proven

Y28 Limited function/disability (Y)   *Z73.6, Z90.7*

excl: sexual dysfunction P07, P08; impotence NOS Y07
criteria: limitation of function/disability due to a problem of the male genital system
             (including breast)
Note: The COOP/WONCA Charts are suitable for documenting the patient's functional
status (see Chapter 8).

Y29 Genital symptom/complaint male, other   *N50.8, N50.9*

Component 7—Diagnosis/diseases

Y70 Syphilis male   *A50 to A53, A65*

incl: syphilis any site
criteria: demonstration of *Treponema pallidum* on microscopy; or positive serologi-
             cal test for syphilis

Y71 Gonorrhoea male   *A54*

incl: gonorrhoea any site   *(cont.)*

criteria: urethral or rectal discharge with Gram-negative intracellular diplococci demonstrated in a patient after a contact with a proven case, or *Neisseria gonorrhoea* cultured

consider: urethritis U72; urethral discharge Y03

Y72 Genital herpes male   *A60*

incl: anogenital herpes

criteria: small vesicles with characteristic appearance and location that evolve to painful ulcers and scabs

Y73 Prostatitis/seminal vesiculitis   *A59.0, N41, N49.0*

criteria: tenderness of prostate/seminal vesicles to palpation, and indications of inflammation in urine test

Y74 Orchitis/epididymitis   *A56.1, N45*

excl: tuberculosis A70; mumps D71; gonococcal orchitis Y71; torsion of testis Y99

criteria: both swelling and tenderness of testes/epididymis, and absence of a specific aetiology (mumps, gonococcal, tuberculosis, trauma, or torsion)

consider: symptom of testis Y05

Y75 Balanitis   *A63.8, B37.4, N48.1*

incl: candidiasis glans penis

excl: scabies S72; male syphilis Y70; male gonorrhoea Y71; male genital herpes Y72

criteria: signs of inflammation of the prepuce/glans penis

Y76 Condylomata acuminata male   *A63.0*

incl: venereal warts, human papilloma virus infection

criteria: characteristic appearance of lesions, or characteristic histological appearance

Y77 Malignant neoplasm prostate   *C61*

criteria: characteristic histological appearance

consider: benign/unspecified neoplasm male genital Y79

Y78 Malignant neoplasm male genital, other   *C50, C60, C62, C63*

incl: carcinoma testis/seminoma, carcinoma breast

excl: carcinoma-in-situ Y79

criteria: characteristic histological appearance

consider: benign/unspecified neoplasm male genital Y79

Y79 Benign/unspecified neoplasm male genital
D05, D07.4 to D07.6, D24, D29, D40, D48.6

incl: benign genital neoplasm, genital neoplasm not specified as benign or malignant/when histology is not available, benign neoplasm male breast, carcinoma-in-situ
excl: prostatic hypertrophy Y85

Y80 Injury male genital
S30.2, S31.2, S31.3, S31.5, S38.0, S38.2, S39.8, S39.9, T28.3, T28.8

incl: circumcision

Y81 Phimosis/redundant prepuce   *N47*

incl: paraphimosis
criteria: for redundant prepuce: excessive length of prepuce, with inability to retract over the glans penis; for phimosis: tightness of prepuce which prevents retraction over the glans penis

Y82 Hypospadias   *Q54*

Y83 Undescended testicle   *Q53*

incl: cryptorchidism
excl: retractile testis Y84
criteria: the testicle has never been observed in the scrotum, and the testicle cannot be manipulated into the scrotum

Y84 Congenital genital anomaly male, other   *Q55, Q56, Q83*

incl: hermaphroditism, retractile testis

Y85 Benign prostatic hypertrophy   *N40*

incl: fibroma, hyperplasia, median bar of prostate, prostatic obstruction, prostatomegaly
criteria: enlarged, smooth, firm prostate demonstrated by palpation/cystoscopy/imaging, with no evidence of prostatic carcinoma
consider: symptom/complaint about urination U01, U02, U03, U04, U05; retention of urine U08

Y86 Hydrocoele   *N43.0 to N43.3*

criteria: non-tender fluctuant swelling surrounding testis or spermatic cord with transillumination of the swelling or imaging evidence
consider: symptom/complaint of scrotum/testis other Y05

Y99 Genital disease male, other

A55, A56.1, A56.3 to A56.8, A57, A58, A63.8, N42.0 to N42.2, N42.8, N42.9, N43.4, N44, N48.0, N48.2, N48.5, N48.6, N48.8, N48.9, N49.1, N49.2, N49.8, N49.9, N50.0, N50.1, N50.8, N50.9, N51, N64.8, N64.9, Z90.7

incl: other disease of male breast, epididymal cyst, spermatocele, torsion of the testis
excl: sexually transmitted disease NOS A78; gynaecomastia Y16; carcinoma male
           breast Y78

Z Social problems

Component 1—Symptoms and complaints

Z01 Poverty/financial problem   *Z59.5 to Z59.9*

Note: Problems with living conditions essentially require the patient's expression of concern about them, with agreement about the existence of the problem and desire for help. Whatever the objective living conditions, patients can consider these as a problem. Labelling these problems requires acknowledgement of absolute differences in living conditions, as well as the individual's perception.

Z02 Food/water problem   *Z58.6, Z59.4*

Note: Problems with living conditions essentially require the patient's expression of concern about them, with agreement about the existence of the problem and desire for help. Whatever the objective living conditions, patients can consider these as a problem. Labelling these problems requires acknowledgement of absolute differences in living conditions, as well as the individual's perception.

Z03 Housing/neighbourhood problem   *Z59.0 to Z59.3, Z59.8, Z59.9*

Note: Problems with living conditions essentially require the patient's expression of concern about them, with agreement about the existence of the problem and desire for help. Whatever the objective living conditions, patients can consider these as a problem. Labelling these problems requires acknowledgement of absolute differences in living conditions, as well as the individual's perception.

Z04 Social cultural problem   *Z60.1 to Z60.9*

incl: illegitimate pregnancy
excl: unwanted pregnancy W79
Note: Problems with living conditions essentially require the patient's expression of concern about them, with agreement about the existence of the problem and desire for help. Whatever the objective living conditions, patients can consider these as a problem. Labelling these problems requires acknowledgement of absolute differences in living conditions, as well as the individual's perception.

Z05 Work problem   *Z56.1 to Z56.7, Z57*

Note: Problems with working conditions essentially require the patient's expression of concern about them, with agreement about the existence of the problem and desire for help. Whatever the objective working conditions, patients can consider these as a problem. Labelling these problems requires acknowledgement of absolute differences in working conditions, as well as the individual's perception.

Z06 Unemployment problem   *Z56.0*

excl: retirement problem P25

Note: Problems with unemployment essentially require the patient's expression of concern about them, with agreement about the existence of the problem and desire for help. Whatever the objective nature of the unemployment, patients can consider this as a problem. Labelling these problems requires acknowledgement of absolute differences in unemployment, as well as the individual's perception.

Z07 Education problem   *Z55*

incl: illiteracy

Note: Problems with education essentially require the patient's expression of concern about them, with agreement about the existence of the problem and desire for help. Whatever the objective education status, patients can consider this as a problem. Labelling these problems requires acknowledgement of absolute differences in education, as well as the individual's perception.

Z08 Social welfare problem   *Z59.7*

Note: Problems with social welfare essentially require the patient's expression of concern about them, with agreement about the existence of the problem and desire for help. Whatever the objective social welfare situation, patients can consider this as a problem. Labelling these problems requires acknowledgement of absolute differences in social welfare, as well as the individual's perception.

Z09 Legal problem   *Z65.0 to Z65.3*

Note: Problems with legal issues essentially require the patient's expression of concern about them, with agreement about the existence of the problem and desire for help. Whatever the objective legal issues, patients can consider these as a problem. Labelling these problems requires acknowledgement of absolute differences in legal issues as well as the individual's perception.

Z10 Health care system problem   *Z64.4, Z75*

Note: Problems with the health care system essentially require the patient's expression of concern about them, with agreement about the existence of the problem and desire for help. Whatever the objective health care system, patients can consider this as a problem.

Labelling these problems requires acknowledgement of absolute differences in the health care system as well as the individual's perception.

Z11 Compliance/being ill problem   *Z75*

incl: poor compliance
Note: The diagnosis of social problems arising due to being ill requires the patient's agreement on the existence of the problem and desire for help.

Z12 Relationship problem with partner   *T74.0, T74.3, Z63.0*

incl: emotional abuse
excl: physical abuse Z25
Note: The diagnosis of problems in the relationship between family partners requires the patient's agreement on the existence of the problem and desire for help.

Z13 Partner's behaviour problem   *Z63.0*

incl: infidelity, physical abuse
Note: The diagnosis of problems arising from the behaviour of a family partner requires the patient's agreement on the existence of the problem and desire for help.

Z14 Partner illness problem   *Z63.6*

Note: The diagnosis of problems arising from one or both family partners being ill requires the patient's agreement on the existence of the problem and desire for help.

Z15 Loss/death of partner problem   *Z63.4, Z63.5*

incl: bereavement, divorce, separation
Note: The diagnosis of problems arising from the loss or death of a family partner requires the patient's agreement on the existence of the problem and desire for help.

Z16 Relationship problem with child   *T74.0, T74.3, Z61, Z62, Z63.8*

incl: child abuse (emotional)
excl: physical abuse Z25
Note: The diagnosis of problems in the relationship with a child requires the patient's agreement on the existence of the problem and desire for help.

Z18 Illness problem with child   *Z63.6*

Note: The diagnosis of problems arising due to a child being ill requires the patient's agreement on the existence of the problem and desire for help.

Z19 Loss/death of child problem   *Z63.4*

Note: The diagnosis of problems arising from the loss or death of a child in the family requires the patient's agreement on the existence of the problem and desire for help.

Z20 Relationship problem, parent/family   *T74.0, Z63.1, Z63.8*

incl: relationship problem with parent/adult sibling/other family member
excl: relationship problem with partner Z12; relationship problem with child Z16; relationship problem with friend Z24
Note: The diagnosis of problems in the relationship between family members requires the patient's agreement on the existence of the problem and desire for help.

Z21 Behaviour problem, parent/family   *Z63.1, Z63.9*

excl: symptom/complaint behaviour of child P22; symptom/complaint behaviour adolescent P23; problem with behaviour partner Z13
Note: The diagnosis of problems arising from the behaviour of a family member requires the patient's agreement on the existence of the problem and desire for help.

Z22 Illness problem, parent/family   *Z63.6, Z63.7*

excl: problem with partner being ill Z14
Note: The diagnosis of problems arising from the illness of a family member requires the patient's agreement on the existence of the problem and desire for help.

Z23 Loss/death of parent/family member problem   *Z63.4*

excl: loss of partner Z15; loss of child Z19
Note: The diagnosis of problems arising from the loss or death of a family member requires the patient's agreement on the existence of the problem and desire for help.

Z24 Relationship problem, friend   *Z63.9*

excl: relationship problem with family member Z20
Note: The diagnosis of problems in the relationship with friends requires the patient's agreement on the existence of the problem and desire for help.

Z25 Assault/harmful event problem   *T74.1, T74.2, T74.8, T74.9, Z65.4, Z65.5*

incl: victim of physical abuse, rape, sexual attack
excl: partner emotional abuse Z12; partner physical abuse Z13; child emotional abuse Z16; physical problems to be coded in appropriate rubric(s) in other Chapters; psychological problems to be coded in Chapter P.
Note: The diagnosis of social problems arising from assaults and other harmful events requires the patient's agreement on the existence of the problem and desire for help.

Z27 fear of a social problem   *Z71.1*

incl: concern about/fear of having a social problem
excl: if the patient has a social problem, code the problem
criteria: fear of a social problem in a patient without the problem

Z28 Limited function/disability (Z)   *Z73.4, Z73.6*

criteria: limitation of function/disability caused by social problems, including isolation/
            living alone/loneliness
Note: The COOP/WONCA Charts are suitable for documenting the patient's functional
status (see Chapter 8).

Z29 Social problem NOS
Z58.0 to Z58.5, Z58.8, Z58.9, Z63.2, Z63.3, Z63.7, Z63.8, Z63.9, Z64.1,
Z65.8, Z65.9, Z72.6, Z72.8, Z72.9, Z73.5, Z73.8, Z73.9, Z76.5

incl: environmental problems, malingering

11 Conversion codes from ICD-10

The relationship between ICPC and ICD-10 is complex. There are some concepts in both that are not represented exactly in the other.[18] However, for most rubrics in each classification one or more corresponding rubrics in the other can be mapped. This has been done in both directions in this book.

Because of these complexities, the conversion of a code from one classification to the other and then re-conversion back again will not necessarily lead back to the same original code, because in each direction there may be several codes to choose from. Exact choices can be made only if the title of the condition is used with the help of a thesaurus. The point of having the code conversions in this book is simply to indicate where the contents of rubrics in each classification overlap.

ICPC-2 to ICD-10

In the tabular list of ICPC-2 rubrics (Chapter 10) each rubric includes all the ICD-10 rubrics to which it relates. Where it relates to all of the three-digit ICD-10 code, this is given; where it relates to only part of the three-digit ICD-10 code, all the relevant four-digit ICD-10 codes are given. However, this does not imply that the ICD-10 codes listed relate only to the ICPC-2 rubric, because some ICD-10 rubrics relate to more than one ICPC-2 rubric, as can be seen by perusing the list of conversion codes from ICD-10 to ICPC-2 in this chapter.

ICD-10 to ICPC-2

In this chapter conversion codes are listed for all ICD-10 three-digit codes, and where not all of a three-digit code maps to the same ICPC-2 code, the conversions for all the four-digit ICD-10 codes are given. Not included are rubrics in Chapter XX of ICD-10, External Causes of Morbidity and Mortality, as ICPC is in general not based on aetiology.

ICD-10	ICPC-2	ICD-10	ICPC-2	ICD-10	ICPC-2	ICD-10	ICPC-2
A00	D70	A06	D70	A17	A70	A23	A78
A01	D70	A07	D70	A18	A70	A24	A78
A02	D70	A08	D70	A19	A70	A25	A78
A03	D70	A09	D73	A20	A78	A26	A78
A04	D70	A15	A70	A21	A78	A27	A78
A05	D70	A16	A70	A22	A78	A28	A78

ICD-10	ICPC-2	ICD-10	ICPC-2	ICD-10	ICPC-2	ICD-10	ICPC-2
A30	A78	A55	Y99	A75	A78	B08.1	S95
A31	A78	A56.0	U72	A77	A78	B08.2	A76
A32.0	A78	A56.0	X92	A78	A78	B08.3	A76
A32.1	A78	A56.1	X92	A79	A78	B08.4	A76
A32.1	N71	A56.1	Y74	A80	N70	B08.5	R74
A32.7	A78	A56.1	Y99	A81	N73	B08.8	A76
A32.8	A78	A56.2	U72	A82	A77	B09	A76
A32.9	A78	A56.2	X92	A83	N71	B15	D72
A33	N72	A56.3	X92	A84	N71	B16	D72
A34	N72	A56.3	Y99	A85.0	N70	B17	D72
A35	N72	A56.4	X92	A85.1	N71	B18	D72
A36	R83	A56.4	Y99	A85.2	N71	B19	D72
A37	R71	A56.8	X92	A85.8	N71	B20	B90
A38	A78	A56.8	Y99	A86	N71	B21	B90
A39.0	N71	A57	X99	A87	N71	B22	B90
A39.1	A78	A57	Y99	A88.0	A76	B23	B90
A39.2	A78	A58	X99	A88.1	H82	B24	B90
A39.3	A78	A58	Y99	A88.8	N73	B25	A77
A39.4	A78	A59.0	U72	A89	N73	B26	D71
A39.5	K70	A59.0	X73	A90	A77	B27	A75
A39.8	A78	A59.0	Y73	A91	A77	B30	F70
A39.9	A78	A59.8	A78	A92	A77	B33.0	A77
A40	A78	A59.9	A78	A93	A77	B33.1	A77
A41	A78	A60	X90	A94	A77	B33.2	K70
A42	A78	A60	Y72	A95	A77	B33.3	A77
A43	A78	A63.0	X91	A96	A77	B33.8	A77
A44	A78	A63.0	Y76	A98	A77	B34	A77
A46	S76	A63.8	X99	A99	A77	B35	S74
A48.0	A78	A63.8	Y75	B00.0	S71	B36	S74
A48.1	R81	A63.8	Y99	B00.1	S71	B37.0	D83
A48.2	A78	A64	A78	B00.2	R74	B37.1	R83
A48.3	A78	A65	X70	B00.2	S71	B37.2	S75
A48.4	A78	A65	Y70	B00.3	N71	B37.3	X72
A48.8	A78	A66	S76	B00.4	N71	B37.4	U72
A49	A78	A67	S76	B00.5	F73	B37.4	X72
A50	X70	A68	A78	B00.7	A77	B37.4	Y75
A50	Y70	A69.0	D83	B00.8	S71	B37.5	N71
A51	X70	A69.1	D83	B00.9	S71	B37.6	K70
A51	Y70	A69.2	A78	B01	A72	B37.7	A78
A52	X70	A69.8	A78	B02	S70	B37.8	A78
A52	Y70	A69.9	A78	B03	A76	B37.9	A78
A53	X70	A70	A78	B04	A76	B38	A78
A53	Y70	A71	F86	B05	A71	B39	A78
A54	X71	A74.0	F70	B06	A74	B40	A78
A54	Y71	A74.8	A78	B07	S03	B41	A78
A55	X99	A74.9	A78	B08.0	A76	B42	A78

ICD-10	ICPC-2	ICD-10	ICPC-2	ICD-10	ICPC-2	ICD-10	ICPC-2
B43	A78	B88.0	S72	C25	D76	C61	Y77
B44	R83	B88.1	S73	C26	D77	C62	Y78
B45	A78	B88.2	S72	C30.0	R85	C63	Y78
B46	A78	B88.3	S73	C30.1	H75	C64	U75
B47	A78	B88.8	S73	C31	R85	C65	U75
B48	A78	B88.9	S73	C32	R85	C66	U77
B49	A78	B89	A78	C33	R84	C67	U76
B50	A73	B90	A70	C34	R84	C68	U77
B51	A73	B91	N70	C37	B74	C69	F74
B52	A73	B92	A78	C38.0	K72	C70	N74
B53	A73	B94.0	F86	C38.1	A79	C71	N74
B54	A73	B94.1	N71	C38.2	A79	C72	N74
B55	A78	B94.2	D97	C38.3	A79	C73	T71
B56	A78	B94.8	A78	C38.4	R85	C74	T73
B57	A78	B94.9	A78	C38.8	A79	C75	T73
B58.0	F73	B95	A78	C39	R85	C76	A79
B58.1	D97	B96	A78	C40	L71	C77	B74
B58.2	N71	B97	A77	C41	L71	C78	A79
B58.3	R83	B99	A78	C43	S77	C79	A79
B58.8	A78	C00	D77	C44	S77	C80	A79
B58.9	A78	C01	D77	C45.0	R85	C81	B72
B59	A78	C02	D77	C45.1	D77	C82	B72
B60	A78	C03	D77	C45.2	K72	C83	B72
B64	A78	C04	D77	C45.7	A79	C84	B72
B65	D96	C05	D77	C45.9	A79	C85	B72
B66	D96	C06	D77	C46.0	S77	C88	B74
B67	D96	C07	D77	C46.1	L71	C90	B74
B68	D96	C08	D77	C46.2	D77	C91	B73
B69	D96	C09	R85	C46.3	B74	C92	B73
B70	D96	C10	R85	C46.7	A79	C93	B73
B71	D96	C11	R85	C46.8	A79	C94	B73
B72	D96	C12	R85	C46.9	A79	C95	B73
B73	D96	C13	R85	C47	N74	C96	B74
B74	D96	C14.0	R85	C48	D77	C97	A79
B75	D96	C14.2	R85	C49	L71	D00	D78
B76	D96	C14.8	D77	C50	X76	D01	D78
B77	D96	C15	D77	C50	Y78	D02	R92
B78	D96	C16	D74	C51	X77	D03	S79
B79	D96	C17	D77	C52	X77	D04	S79
B80	D96	C18	D75	C53	X75	D05	X81
B81	D96	C19	D75	C54	X77	D05	Y79
B82	D96	C20	D75	C55	X77	D06	X81
B83	D96	C21	D75	C56	X77	D07.0	X81
B85	S73	C22	D77	C57	X77	D07.1	X81
B86	S72	C23	D77	C58	W72	D07.2	X81
B87	S73	C24	D77	C60	Y78	D07.3	X81

ICD-10	ICPC-2	ICD-10	ICPC-2	ICD-10	ICPC-2	ICD-10	ICPC-2
D07.4	Y79	D36.1	N75	D61.2	A86	E06.9	T99
D07.5	Y79	D36.7	A99	D61.3	B82	E07	T99
D07.6	Y79	D36.9	A99	D61.8	B82	E10	T89
D09.0	U79	D37	D78	D61.9	B82	E11	T90
D09.1	U79	D38.0	R92	D62	B82	E12	T90
D09.2	F74	D38.1	R92	D63	B82	E13	T90
D09.3	T73	D38.2	R92	D64.0	B79	E14	T90
D09.7	A79	D38.3	R92	D64.1	B82	E15	T87
D09.9	A79	D38.4	R92	D64.2	A85	E16.0	T87
D10	D78	D38.5	H75	D64.2	A86	E16.1	T87
D11	D78	D38.5	R92	D64.3	B82	E16.2	T87
D12	D78	D38.6	R92	D64.4	B79	E16.3	T87
D13	D78	D39	X81	D64.8	B82	E16.4	D86
D14.0	H75	D40	Y79	D64.9	B82	E16.8	T99
D14.0	R86	D41	U79	D65	B83	E16.9	T87
D14.1	R86	D42	N76	D66	B83	E20	T99
D14.2	R86	D43	N76	D67	B83	E21	T99
D14.3	R86	D44	T73	D68	B83	E22	T99
D14.4	R86	D45	B75	D69	B83	E23	T99
D15.0	B75	D46	B82	D70	B84	E24	T99
D15.1	K72	D47	B75	D71	B84	E25	T99
D15.2	K72	D48.0	L97	D72	B84	E26	T99
D15.7	A99	D48.1	H75	D73	B99	E27	T99
D15.9	A99	D48.1	L97	D74	B99	E28	T99
D16	L97	D48.2	N76	D75	B99	E29	T99
D17	S78	D48.3	D78	D76	B99	E30	T99
D18	S81	D48.4	D78	D77	B99	E31	T99
D19	R86	D48.5	H75	D80	B99	E32	T99
D20	D78	D48.5	S79	D81	B99	E34.0	T99
D21	L97	D48.6	X81	D82	B99	E34.1	T99
D22	S82	D48.6	Y79	D83	B99	E34.2	T99
D23	S79	D48.7	F74	D84	B99	E34.3	T10
D24	X79	D48.7	K72	D86	B99	E34.4	T99
D24	Y79	D48.9	A99	D89	B99	E34.5	T99
D25	X78	D50	B80	E00	T80	E34.8	T99
D26	X80	D51	B81	E01	T86	E34.9	T99
D27	X80	D52	B81	E02	T86	E35	T99
D28	X80	D53	B82	E03	T86	E40	T91
D29	Y79	D55	B82	E04	T81	E41	T91
D30	U78	D56	B78	E05	T85	E42	T91
D31	F74	D57	B78	E06.0	T70	E43	T91
D32	N75	D58	B78	E06.1	T99	E44	T91
D33	N75	D59	B82	E06.2	T99	E45	T91
D34	T72	D60	B82	E06.3	T99	E46	T91
D35	T73	D61.0	B79	E06.4	T99	E50	T91
D36.0	B75	D61.1	A85	E06.5	T99	E51.1	T91

ICD-10	ICPC-2	ICD-10	ICPC-2	ICD-10	ICPC-2	ICD-10	ICPC-2
E51.2	N99	F09	P71	F41.9	P74	F63.2	P80
E51.8	T91	F10.0	P16	F42	P79	F63.3	P29
E51.9	T91	F10.1	P15	F43.0	P02	F63.8	P80
E52	T91	F10.2	P15	F43.1	P82	F63.9	P80
E53	T91	F10.3	P15	F43.2	P02	F64	P09
E54	T91	F10.4	P15	F43.8	P02	F65	P09
E55	T91	F10.5	P15	F43.9	P02	F66	P09
E56	T91	F10.6	P15	F44	P75	F68	P80
E58	T91	F10.7	P15	F45.0	P75	F69	P80
E59	T91	F10.8	P15	F45.1	P75	F70	P85
E60	T91	F10.9	P15	F45.2	P75	F71	P85
E61	T91	F11	P19	F48.0	P78	F72	P85
E63	T91	F12	P19	F48.1	P99	F73	P85
E64	T91	F13	P18	F48.8	P99	F78	P85
E65	T99	F13	P19	F48.9	P99	F79	P85
E66	T82	F14	P19	F50.0	P86	F80	P24
E66	T83	F15	P19	F50.1	P86	F81	P24
E67	T99	F16	P19	F50.2	P86	F82	P24
E68	T99	F17	P17	F50.3	P86	F83	P24
E70	T99	F18	P19	F50.4	P86	F84	P99
E71	T99	F19	P18	F50.5	D10	F88	P99
E72	T99	F19	P19	F50.8	P29	F89	P99
E73	T99	F20	P72	F50.9	P29	F90	P81
E74	T99	F21	P72	F51	P06	F91	P22
E75	T99	F22	P72	F52.0	P07	F91	P23
E76	T99	F23	P98	F52.1	P08	F92	P22
E77	T99	F24	P72	F52.2	P08	F92	P23
E78	T93	F25	P72	F52.3	P08	F93	P22
E79	T99	F28	P72	F52.4	P08	F94	P22
E80	T99	F29	P98	F52.5	P08	F94	P23
E83	T99	F30	P73	F52.6	P08	F95	P10
E84	T99	F31	P73	F52.7	P08	F98.0	P12
E85	T99	F32	P76	F52.8	P08	F98.1	P13
E86	T11	F33	P76	F52.9	P08	F98.2	P11
E87	T99	F34.0	P73	F53.0	P76	F98.3	P11
E88	T99	F34.1	P76	F53.1	P98	F98.4	P10
E89	A87	F34.8	P76	F53.8	P99	F98.5	P10
E90	T99	F34.9	P76	F53.9	P99	F98.6	P10
F00	P70	F38	P76	F54	P99	F98.8	P22
F01	P70	F39	P76	F55	P18	F98.8	P23
F02	P70	F40	P79	F59	P99	F98.8	P29
F03	P70	F41.0	P74	F60	P80	F98.9	P22
F04	P71	F41.1	P74	F61	P80	F98.9	P23
F05	P71	F41.2	P76	F62	P80	F98.9	P29
F06	P71	F41.3	P74	F63.0	P80	F99	P99
F07	P71	F41.8	P74	F63.1	P80	G00	N71

ICD-10	ICPC-2	ICD-10	ICPC-2	ICD-10	ICPC-2	ICD-10	ICPC-2
G01	N71	G44.4	A85	G93.6	N99	H10.2	F70
G02	N71	G44.8	N01	G93.7	N99	H10.3	F70
G03	N71	G45	K89	G93.8	N99	H10.4	F70
G04	N71	G46	K90	G93.9	N99	H10.5	F70
G05	N71	G47	P06	G94	N99	H10.8	F70
G06	N73	G50.0	N92	G95	N99	H10.9	F70
G07	N73	G50.1	N03	G96	N99	H11.0	F99
G08	N73	G50.8	N92	G97	A87	H11.1	F99
G09	N73	G50.9	N92	G98	N18	H11.2	F99
G10	N99	G51	N91	G98	N99	H11.3	F75
G11	N99	G52	N99	G99	N99	H11.4	F99
G12	N99	G53	N91	H00	F72	H11.8	F99
G13	N99	G54	N94	H01	F72	H11.9	F99
G20	N87	G55	N94	H02.0	F99	H13	F70
G21	N87	G56.0	N93	H02.1	F99	H15	F99
G22	N87	G56.1	N94	H02.2	F16	H16.0	F85
G23	N99	G56.2	N94	H02.3	F16	H16.1	F73
G24	N99	G56.3	N94	H02.4	F16	H16.1	F79
G25.0	N08	G56.4	N94	H02.5	F16	H16.2	F73
G25.1	N08	G56.8	N94	H02.6	F16	H16.3	F73
G25.2	N08	G56.9	N94	H02.7	F16	H16.4	F73
G25.3	N08	G57	N94	H02.8	F16	H16.8	F73
G25.4	N08	G58	N94	H02.8	F99	H16.9	F73
G25.5	N08	G59	N94	H02.9	F16	H17	F99
G25.6	N08	G60	N94	H02.9	F99	H18	F99
G25.8	N04	G61	N94	H03	F73	H19	F85
G25.8	N08	G62	N94	H04.0	F99	H20	F73
G25.9	N08	G63	N94	H04.1	F99	H21	F73
G26	N99	G64	N94	H04.2	F03	H22	F73
G30	P70	G70	N99	H04.3	F73	H25	F92
G31.0	N99	G71	N99	H04.4	F73	H26	F92
G31.1	N99	G72	N99	H04.5	F99	H27	F99
G31.2	P15	G73	N99	H04.6	F99	H28	F92
G31.8	N99	G80	N99	H04.8	F99	H30	F73
G31.9	N99	G81	N99	H04.9	F99	H31	F99
G32	N99	G82	N99	H05.0	F73	H32	F73
G35	N86	G83	N99	H05.1	F73	H33	F82
G36	N99	G90	N99	H05.2	F99	H34	F99
G37	N99	G91	N99	H05.3	F99	H35.0	F83
G40	N88	G92	N99	H05.4	F99	H35.1	F83
G41	N88	G93.0	N99	H05.5	F99	H35.2	F83
G43	N89	G93.1	N99	H05.8	F99	H35.3	F84
G44.0	N90	G93.2	N99	H05.9	F99	H35.4	F83
G44.1	N89	G93.3	A04	H06	F99	H35.5	F99
G44.2	N95	G93.4	N99	H10.0	F70	H35.6	F99
G44.3	N01	G93.5	N99	H10.1	F71	H35.7	F99

ICD-10	ICPC-2	ICD-10	ICPC-2	ICD-10	ICPC-2	ICD-10	ICPC-2
H35.8	F99	H57.8	F02	H83.8	H99	I30	K70
H35.9	F99	H57.8	F13	H83.9	H99	I31	K84
H36	F83	H57.8	F15	H90	H86	I32	K70
H40	F93	H57.8	F75	H91.0	H86	I33	K70
H42	F93	H57.8	F99	H91.1	H84	I34	K83
H43	F99	H57.9	F29	H91.2	H86	I35	K83
H44.0	F99	H58	F99	H91.3	H86	I36	K83
H44.1	F99	H59	A87	H91.8	H86	I37	K83
H44.2	F99	H60	H70	H91.9	H86	I38	K70
H44.3	F99	H61.0	H99	H92.0	H01	I39	K70
H44.4	F99	H61.1	H99	H92.1	H04	I40	K70
H44.5	F99	H61.2	H81	H92.2	H05	I41	K70
H44.6	F79	H61.3	H99	H93.0	H99	I42.0	K84
H44.7	F79	H61.8	H99	H93.1	H03	I42.1	K84
H44.8	F99	H61.9	H99	H93.2	H02	I42.2	K84
H44.9	F99	H62	H70	H93.3	H99	I42.3	K84
H45	F99	H65	H72	H93.8	H13	I42.4	K73
H46	F99	H66.0	H71	H93.8	H99	I42.5	K84
H47	F99	H66.1	H74	H93.9	H29	I42.6	K84
H48	F99	H66.2	H74	H94	H99	I42.7	K84
H49	F95	H66.3	H74	H95	A87	I42.8	K84
H50	F95	H66.4	H71	I00	K71	I42.9	K84
H51	F95	H66.9	H71	I01	K71	I43	K84
H52	F91	H67	H71	I02	K71	I44	K84
H53.0	F99	H68	H73	I05	K71	I45	K84
H53.1	F04	H69	H73	I06	K71	I46	K84
H53.1	F05	H70.0	H71	I07	K71	I47	K79
H53.2	F05	H70.1	H74	I08	K71	I48	K78
H53.3	F05	H70.2	H74	I09	K71	I49	K80
H53.4	F99	H70.8	H74	I10	K86	I50	K77
H53.5	F99	H70.9	H74	I11	K87	I51	K84
H53.6	F99	H71	H74	I12	K87	I52	K84
H53.8	F05	H72	H77	I13	K87	I60	K90
H53.8	F99	H73.0	H71	I15	K87	I61	K90
H53.9	F05	H73.1	H74	I20	K74	I62	K90
H54.0	F94	H73.8	H99	I21	K75	I63	K90
H54.1	F94	H73.9	H99	I22	K75	I64	K90
H54.2	F94	H74	H99	I23	K75	I65	K91
H54.3	F94	H75	H74	I24.0	K74	I66	K91
H54.4	F28	H80	H83	I24.1	K75	I67.0	K91
H54.5	F28	H81	H82	I24.8	K74	I67.1	K91
H54.6	F28	H82	H82	I24.9	K74	I67.2	K91
H54.7	F05	H83.0	H82	I25	K76	I67.3	K91
H55	F14	H83.1	H99	I26	K93	I67.4	K87
H57.0	F99	H83.2	H99	I27	K82	I67.5	K91
H57.1	F01	H83.3	H85	I28	K82	I67.6	K91

ICD-10	ICPC-2	ICD-10	ICPC-2	ICD-10	ICPC-2	ICD-10	ICPC-2
I67.7	K91	J01	R75	J41	R79	K03.1	D82
I67.8	K91	J02.0	R72	J42	R79	K03.2	D82
I67.9	K91	J02.8	R74	J43	R95	K03.3	D82
I68	K91	J02.9	R74	J44	R95	K03.4	D82
I69	K91	J03.0	R72	J45	R96	K03.5	D82
I70	K92	J03.8	R76	J46	R96	K03.6	D82
I71	K99	J03.9	R76	J47	R99	K03.7	D82
I72	K99	J04	R77	J60	R99	K03.8	D29
I73	K92	J05.0	R77	J61	R99	K03.8	D82
I74	K92	J05.1	R83	J62	R99	K03.9	D82
I77	K99	J06	R74	J63	R99	K04	D82
I78.0	K99	J10.0	R81	J64	R99	K05	D82
I78.1	K06	J10.1	R80	J65	R99	K06	D82
I78.8	K99	J10.8	R80	J66	R99	K07.0	D82
I78.9	K99	J11.0	R81	J67	R99	K07.1	D82
I79	K99	J11.1	R80	J68	R99	K07.2	D82
I80	K94	J11.8	R80	J69	R99	K07.3	D82
I81	K94	J12	R81	J70	R99	K07.4	D82
I82	K94	J13	R81	J80	R99	K07.5	D82
I83.0	S97	J14	R81	J81	R99	K07.6	D82
I83.1	K95	J15	R81	J82	R99	K07.6	L07
I83.2	S97	J16	R81	J84	R99	K07.8	D82
I83.9	K95	J17	R81	J85	R83	K07.9	D82
I84	K96	J18	R81	J86	R83	K08.0	D82
I85	K99	J20	R78	J90	R82	K08.1	D82
I86	K99	J21	R78	J91	R82	K08.2	D82
I87.0	K94	J22	R78	J92	R99	K08.3	D82
I87.1	K99	J30	R97	J93	R99	K08.8	D19
I87.2	K95	J31	R83	J94	R82	K08.8	D82
I87.8	K06	J32	R75	J95	A87	K08.9	D82
I87.8	K94	J33	R99	J96	R99	K09	D82
I87.9	K99	J34.0	R73	J98	R99	K10	D82
I88	B71	J34.1	R99	J99	R99	K11	D83
I89.0	K99	J34.2	R99	K00.0	D82	K12	D83
I89.1	B99	J34.3	R99	K00.1	D82	K13.0	D83
I89.8	B99	J34.8	R07	K00.2	D82	K13.1	D20
I89.9	B99	J34.8	R08	K00.3	D82	K13.2	D83
I95.0	K88	J34.8	R09	K00.4	D82	K13.3	D83
I95.1	K88	J34.8	R90	K00.5	D82	K13.4	D83
I95.2	A85	J34.8	R99	K00.6	D82	K13.5	D83
I95.8	K88	J35	R90	K00.7	D19	K13.6	D83
I95.9	K88	J36	R76	K00.8	D82	K13.7	D20
I97	A87	J37	R83	K00.9	D82	K13.7	D83
I98	K99	J38	R99	K01	D82	K14.0	D83
I99	K99	J39	R99	K02	D82	K14.1	D83
J00	R74	J40	R78	K03.0	D82	K14.2	D83

ICD-10	ICPC-2	ICD-10	ICPC-2	ICD-10	ICPC-2	ICD-10	ICPC-2
K14.3	D83	K52.9	D99	K82	D98	L27.1	A85
K14.4	D83	K55	D99	K83	D98	L27.2	S88
K14.5	D20	K56.0	D99	K85	D99	L27.8	S88
K14.6	D20	K56.1	D99	K86	D99	L27.9	S88
K14.8	D20	K56.2	D99	K87.0	D98	L28	S99
K14.8	D83	K56.3	D99	K87.1	D99	L29.0	D05
K14.9	D20	K56.4	D12	K90	D99	L29.1	Y05
K14.9	D83	K56.5	D99	K91.0	A87	L29.2	X16
K20	D84	K56.6	D99	K91.1	D99	L29.3	D05
K21	D84	K56.7	D99	K91.2	D99	L29.8	S02
K22	D84	K57	D92	K91.3	A87	L29.9	S02
K23	D84	K58	D93	K91.4	A89	L30.0	S88
K25	D86	K59.0	D12	K91.5	D99	L30.1	S92
K26	D85	K59.1	D11	K91.8	D99	L30.2	S99
K27	D86	K59.2	D99	K91.9	D99	L30.3	S88
K28	D86	K59.3	D99	K92.0	D14	L30.4	S88
K29	D87	K59.4	D04	K92.1	D15	L30.5	S99
K30	D07	K59.8	D99	K92.2	D99	L30.8	S88
K31.0	D87	K59.9	D99	K92.8	D99	L30.9	S88
K31.1	D87	K60	D95	K92.9	D99	L40	S91
K31.2	D87	K61	D95	K93	D99	L41	S99
K31.3	D87	K62.0	D78	L00	S84	L42	S90
K31.4	D87	K62.1	D78	L01	S84	L43	S99
K31.5	D87	K62.2	D99	L02	S10	L44	S99
K31.6	D87	K62.3	D99	L03.0	S09	L45	S99
K31.7	D78	K62.4	D99	L03.1	S76	L50	S98
K31.8	D87	K62.5	D16	L03.2	S76	L51	S99
K31.9	D87	K62.6	D99	L03.3	S76	L52	S99
K35	D88	K62.7	D99	L03.8	S76	L53.0	S99
K36	D88	K62.8	D04	L03.9	S76	L53.1	S99
K37	D88	K62.8	D99	L04	B70	L53.2	S99
K38	D99	K62.9	D99	L05	S85	L53.3	S99
K40	D89	K63	D99	L08	S76	L53.8	S99
K41	D91	K65	D99	L10	S99	L53.9	S06
K42	D91	K66	D99	L11	S99	L53.9	S07
K43	D91	K67	D99	L12	S99	L54	S99
K44	D90	K70	D97	L13	S99	L55	S80
K45	D91	K71	D97	L14	S99	L56	S80
K46	D91	K72	D97	L20	S87	L57	S80
K50	D94	K73	D97	L21	S86	L58	S80
K51	D94	K74	D97	L22	S89	L59	S80
K52.0	D94	K75	D97	L23	S88	L60.0	S94
K52.1	D99	K76	D97	L24	S88	L60.1	S22
K52.2	D99	K77	D97	L25	S88	L60.2	S99
K52.8	D99	K80	D98	L26	S99	L60.3	S99
K52.9	D11	K81	D98	L27.0	A85	L60.4	S22

ICD-10	ICPC-2	ICD-10	ICPC-2	ICD-10	ICPC-2	ICD-10	ICPC-2
L60.5	S22	L93	S99	M25.1	L99	M43.0	L84
L60.8	S99	L94	S99	M25.2	L99	M43.1	L83
L60.9	S22	L95	S99	M25.3	L99	M43.1	L84
L62	S22	L97	S97	M25.4	L08	M43.2	L99
L63	S23	L98.0	S76	M25.4	L10	M43.3	L83
L64	S23	L98.1	S99	M25.4	L11	M43.4	L83
L65	S23	L98.2	S99	M25.4	L12	M43.5	L83
L66	S23	L98.3	S99	M25.4	L13	M43.5	L84
L67	S24	L98.4	S97	M25.4	L15	M43.6	L83
L68	S24	L98.5	S99	M25.4	L16	M43.8	L85
L70	S96	L98.6	S99	M25.4	L17	M43.9	L85
L71	S99	L98.8	S99	M25.4	L20	M45	L88
L72.0	S99	L98.9	S99	M25.5	L08	M46.0	L83
L72.1	S93	L99	S99	M25.5	L10	M46.0	L84
L72.2	S99	M00	L70	M25.5	L11	M46.1	L84
L72.8	S99	M01	L70	M25.5	L12	M46.2	L70
L72.9	S99	M02	L99	M25.5	L13	M46.3	L70
L73.0	S99	M03	L99	M25.5	L15	M46.4	L70
L73.1	S99	M05	L88	M25.5	L16	M46.5	L70
L73.2	S92	M06	L88	M25.5	L17	M46.8	L84
L73.8	S99	M07	L99	M25.5	L20	M46.9	L84
L73.9	S99	M08	L88	M25.6	L08	M47.0	L84
L74	S92	M09	L99	M25.6	L10	M47.1	L83
L75	S92	M10	T92	M25.6	L11	M47.1	L86
L80	S99	M11	T99	M25.6	L12	M47.2	L83
L81.0	S08	M12	L99	M25.6	L13	M47.2	L86
L81.1	S08	M13	L91	M25.6	L15	M47.8	L83
L81.2	S08	M14	L99	M25.6	L16	M47.8	L84
L81.3	S08	M15	L91	M25.6	L17	M47.9	L83
L81.4	S99	M16	L89	M25.6	L20	M47.9	L84
L81.5	S99	M17	L90	M25.7	L99	M48	L83
L81.6	S99	M18	L91	M25.8	L20	M48	L84
L81.7	S99	M19	L91	M25.8	L99	M49	L99
L81.8	S99	M19	L92	M25.9	L20	M50	L83
L81.9	S99	M20	L98	M25.9	L99	M51.0	L86
L82	S99	M21	L98	M30	K99	M51.1	L86
L83	S99	M22.0	L80	M31	K99	M51.2	L84
L84	S20	M22.1	L80	M32	L99	M51.2	L86
L85	S99	M22.2	L99	M33	L99	M51.3	L84
L86	S99	M22.3	L99	M34	L99	M51.3	L86
L87	S99	M22.4	L99	M35	L99	M51.4	L84
L88	S99	M22.8	L99	M36	L99	M51.4	L86
L89	S97	M22.9	L99	M40	L85	M51.8	L84
L90	S99	M23	L99	M41	L85	M51.8	L86
L91	S99	M24	L99	M42	L94	M51.9	L84
L92	S99	M25.0	L99	M43.0	L83	M51.9	L86

ICD-10	ICPC-2	*ICD-10*	ICPC-2	*ICD-10*	ICPC-2	*ICD-10*	ICPC-2
M53.0	L83	*M67.2*	L99	*M84*	L99	*N31*	U99
M53.1	L83	*M67.3*	L87	*M85*	L99	*N32*	U99
M53.2	L84	*M67.4*	L87	*M86*	L70	*N33*	U99
M53.3	L03	*M67.8*	L99	*M87*	L99	*N34*	U72
M53.3	L84	*M67.9*	L99	*M88*	L99	*N35*	U99
M53.8	L83	*M68*	L99	*M89*	L99	*N36*	U99
M53.8	L84	*M70*	L87	*M90*	L99	*N37*	U99
M53.9	L83	*M71.0*	L70	*M91*	L94	*N39.0*	U71
M53.9	L84	*M71.1*	L70	*M92*	L94	*N39.1*	U98
M54.0	L01	*M71.2*	L87	*M93*	L94	*N39.2*	U90
M54.0	L02	*M71.3*	L87	*M94*	L99	*N39.3*	U04
M54.0	L03	*M71.4*	L87	*M95*	L99	*N39.4*	U04
M54.1	L99	*M71.5*	L87	*M96*	A87	*N39.8*	U99
M54.2	L01	*M71.8*	L87	*M99*	L99	*N39.9*	U99
M54.3	L86	*M71.9*	L87	*N00*	U88	*N40*	Y85
M54.4	L86	*M72*	L87	*N01*	U88	*N41*	Y73
M54.5	L03	*M73*	L99	*N02*	U06	*N42.0*	Y99
M54.6	L02	*M75*	L92	*N03*	U88	*N42.1*	Y99
M54.8	L02	*M76*	L87	*N04*	U88	*N42.2*	Y99
M54.9	L02	*M77.0*	L87	*N05*	U88	*N42.8*	Y06
M60.0	L70	*M77.1*	L93	*N06*	U99	*N42.8*	Y99
M60.1	L18	*M77.2*	L87	*N07*	U88	*N42.9*	Y06
M60.2	L18	*M77.3*	L87	*N08*	U88	*N42.9*	Y99
M60.8	L18	*M77.4*	L17	*N10*	U70	*N43.0*	Y86
M60.9	L18	*M77.5*	L17	*N11*	U70	*N43.1*	Y86
M61	L99	*M77.8*	L87	*N12*	U70	*N43.2*	Y86
M62.0	L99	*M77.9*	L87	*N13*	U99	*N43.3*	Y86
M62.1	L99	*M79.0*	L18	*N14*	U88	*N43.4*	Y99
M62.2	L99	*M79.1*	L18	*N15.0*	U88	*N44*	Y99
M62.3	L99	*M79.2*	N29	*N15.1*	U70	*N45*	Y74
M62.4	L99	*M79.2*	N94	*N15.8*	U88	*N46*	Y10
M62.5	L19	*M79.2*	N99	*N15.9*	U70	*N47*	Y81
M62.6	L19	*M79.3*	L18	*N16*	U88	*N48.0*	Y99
M62.8	L99	*M79.4*	L99	*N17*	U99	*N48.1*	Y75
M62.9	L99	*M79.5*	L81	*N18*	U99	*N48.2*	Y99
M63	L99	*M79.6*	L09	*N19*	U99	*N48.3*	Y08
M65.0	L70	*M79.6*	L12	*N20*	U95	*N48.4*	Y07
M65.1	L70	*M79.6*	L14	*N21*	U95	*N48.5*	Y99
M65.2	L87	*M79.6*	L17	*N22*	U95	*N48.6*	Y99
M65.3	L87	*M79.6*	L18	*N23*	U14	*N48.8*	Y01
M65.4	L87	*M79.8*	L99	*N25*	U99	*N48.8*	Y04
M65.8	L87	*M79.9*	L19	*N26*	U99	*N48.8*	Y08
M65.9	L87	*M80*	L95	*N27*	U99	*N48.8*	Y99
M66	L99	*M81*	L95	*N28*	U99	*N48.9*	Y04
M67.0	L99	*M82*	L95	*N29*	U99	*N48.9*	Y99
M67.1	L99	*M83*	T99	*N30*	U71	*N49.0*	Y73

ICD-10	ICPC-2	ICD-10	ICPC-2	ICD-10	ICPC-2	ICD-10	ICPC-2
N49.1	Y99	N74.8	X74	N92.5	X07	O16	W81
N49.2	Y99	N75	X99	N92.6	X07	O20	W03
N49.8	Y99	N76	X84	N93.0	X13	O21	W05
N49.9	Y99	N77	X84	N93.8	X08	O22	W99
N50.0	Y99	N80	X99	N93.9	X08	O23	W71
N50.1	Y99	N81	X87	N94.0	X03	O24.0	W84
N50.8	Y02	N82	X99	N94.1	X04	O24.1	W84
N50.8	Y05	N83	X99	N94.2	X04	O24.2	W84
N50.8	Y29	N84.0	X99	N94.3	X89	O24.3	W84
N50.8	Y99	N84.1	X85	N94.4	X02	O24.4	W85
N50.9	Y05	N84.2	X99	N94.5	X02	O24.9	W84
N50.9	Y29	N84.3	X99	N94.6	X02	O25	W84
N50.9	Y99	N84.8	X99	N94.8	X01	O26	W29
N51	Y99	N84.9	X99	N94.8	X09	O26	W99
N60	X88	N85	X99	N94.8	X17	O28	W99
N61	X21	N86	X85	N94.8	X29	O29	A87
N61	X99	N87	X86	N94.8	X99	O30	W84
N62	X21	N88	X85	N94.9	X09	O31	W84
N62	Y16	N89.0	X99	N94.9	X17	O32	W84
N63	X19	N89.1	X99	N94.9	X29	O33	W84
N63	Y16	N89.2	X99	N94.9	X99	O34	W84
N64.0	X20	N89.3	X99	N95.0	X12	O35	W84
N64.1	X99	N89.4	X99	N95.1	X11	O36	W84
N64.2	X99	N89.5	X99	N95.2	X11	O40	W84
N64.3	X21	N89.6	X99	N95.3	X11	O41.0	W99
N64.4	X18	N89.7	X99	N95.8	X11	O41.1	W71
N64.5	X20	N89.8	X14	N95.9	X11	O41.8	W99
N64.5	X21	N89.8	X15	N96	X99	O41.9	W99
N64.5	Y16	N89.9	X15	N97	W15	O42	W92
N64.8	X21	N90.0	X99	N98	X99	O42	W93
N64.8	X88	N90.1	X99	N99	A87	O43	W84
N64.8	X99	N90.2	X99	O00	W80	O44	W84
N64.8	Y99	N90.3	X99	O01	W73	O45	W92
N64.9	X21	N90.4	X99	O02	W82	O45	W93
N64.9	X88	N90.5	X99	O03	W82	O46	W03
N64.9	X99	N90.6	X99	O04	W83	O47	W99
N64.9	Y99	N90.7	X99	O05	W82	O48	W99
N70	X74	N90.8	X99	O06	W82	O60	W92
N71	X74	N90.9	X16	O07	W99	O60	W93
N72	X85	N91	X05	O08	W99	O61	W92
N73	X74	N92.0	X06	O10	W81	O61	W93
N74.0	A70	N92.0	X07	O11	W81	O62	W92
N74.1	A70	N92.1	X07	O12	W81	O62	W93
N74.2	X70	N92.2	X06	O13	W81	O63	W92
N74.3	X71	N92.3	X08	O14	W81	O63	W93
N74.4	X92	N92.4	X06	O15	W81	O64	W92

ICD-10	ICPC-2	*ICD-10*	ICPC-2	*ICD-10*	ICPC-2	*ICD-10*	ICPC-2
O64	W93	O85	W70	P05	A94	P83	A94
O65	W92	O86.0	A87	P07	A93	P90	A94
O65	W93	O86.1	W70	P08	A94	P91	A94
O66	W92	O86.2	W71	P10	A94	P92	A94
O66	W93	O86.3	W70	P11	A94	P93	A94
O67	W92	O86.4	W71	P12	A94	P94	A94
O67	W93	O86.8	W71	P13	A94	P95	A95
O68	W92	O87	W96	P14	A94	P96	A94
O68	W93	O88	W99	P15	A94	Q00	N85
O69	W92	O89	A87	P20	A94	Q01	N85
O69	W93	O90.0	A87	P21	A94	Q02	N85
O70	W92	O90.1	A87	P22	A94	Q03	N85
O70	W93	O90.2	A87	P23	A94	Q04	N85
O71	W92	O90.3	K84	P24	A94	Q05	N85
O71	W93	O90.4	W96	P25	A94	Q06	N85
O72	W17	O90.5	W99	P26	A94	Q07	N85
O73	W92	O90.8	W96	P27	A94	Q10.0	F81
O73	W93	O90.9	W18	P28	A94	Q10.1	F81
O74	A87	O90.9	W96	P29	A94	Q10.2	F81
O75.0	W92	O91	W94	P35	A94	Q10.3	F81
O75.0	W93	O92.0	W95	P36	A94	Q10.4	F81
O75.1	W92	O92.1	W95	P37	A94	Q10.5	F80
O75.1	W93	O92.2	W95	P38	A94	Q10.6	F81
O75.2	W71	O92.3	W95	P39	A94	Q10.7	F81
O75.3	W71	O92.4	W95	P50	A94	Q11	F81
O75.4	W92	O92.5	W19	P51	A94	Q12	F81
O75.4	W93	O92.6	W19	P52	A94	Q13	F81
O75.5	W92	O92.7	W19	P53	A94	Q14	F81
O75.5	W93	O95	W99	P54	A94	Q15	F81
O75.6	W92	O96	W99	P55	A94	Q16	H80
O75.6	W93	O97	W99	P56	A94	Q17	H80
O75.7	W92	O98	W71	P57	A94	Q18	D81
O75.7	W93	O99.0	W84	P58	A94	Q20	K73
O75.8	W92	O99.1	W84	P59	A94	Q21	K73
O75.8	W93	O99.2	W84	P60	A94	Q22	K73
O75.9	W92	O99.3	W84	P61	A94	Q23	K73
O75.9	W93	O99.4	W84	P70	A94	Q24	K73
O80	W90	O99.5	W84	P71	A94	Q25	K73
O81	W92	O99.6	W84	P72	A94	Q26	K73
O81	W93	O99.7	W84	P74	A94	Q27	K73
O82	W92	O99.8	W76	P75	A94	Q28	K73
O82	W93	P00	A94	P76	A94	Q30	R89
O83	W92	P01	A94	P77	A94	Q31	R89
O83	W93	P02	A94	P78	A94	Q32	R89
O84	W92	P03	A94	P80	A94	Q33	R89
O84	W93	P04	A94	P81	A94	Q34	R89

ICD-10	ICPC-2	ICD-10	ICPC-2	ICD-10	ICPC-2	ICD-10	ICPC-2
Q35	D81	Q86	A90	R07.2	K02	R20.3	N06
Q36	D81	Q87	A90	R07.3	L04	R20.8	N06
Q37	D81	Q89.0	B79	R07.4	A11	R20.8	S01
Q38	D81	Q89.1	T80	R09.0	R29	R21	S06
Q39	D81	Q89.2	T78	R09.1	R82	R21	S07
Q40	D81	Q89.2	T80	R09.2	R29	R22.0	S04
Q41	D81	Q89.3	A90	R09.3	R25	R22.1	S04
Q42	D81	Q89.4	A90	R09.8	K03	R22.2	S04
Q43	D81	Q89.7	A90	R09.8	K29	R22.3	S04
Q44	D81	Q89.8	B79	R09.8	K81	R22.4	S04
Q45	D81	Q89.9	A90	R09.8	R21	R22.7	S05
Q50	X83	Q90	A90	R09.8	R29	R22.9	S04
Q51	X83	Q91	A90	R10.0	D01	R23.0	S08
Q52	X83	Q92	A90	R10.1	D02	R23.1	S08
Q53	Y83	Q93	A90	R10.1	D06	R23.2	S08
Q54	Y82	Q95	A90	R10.2	D04	R23.3	S29
Q55	Y84	Q96	A90	R10.2	D06	R23.4	S21
Q56	X83	Q97	A90	R10.2	Y02	R23.8	S04
Q56	Y84	Q98	A90	R10.3	D04	R23.8	S05
Q60	U85	Q99	A90	R10.3	D06	R23.8	S08
Q61	U85	R00.0	K04	R10.4	D01	R23.8	S29
Q62	U85	R00.1	K04	R11	D09	R25.0	N08
Q63	U85	R00.2	K04	R11	D10	R25.1	N08
Q64	U85	R00.8	K05	R11	D29	R25.2	L07
Q65	L82	R01	K81	R12	D03	R25.2	L09
Q66	L82	R02	K92	R13	D21	R25.2	L12
Q67	L82	R03.0	K85	R14	D08	R25.2	L14
Q68	L82	R03.1	K29	R15	D17	R25.2	L17
Q69	L82	R04.0	R06	R16.0	D23	R25.2	L18
Q70	L82	R04.1	R29	R16.1	B87	R25.3	N08
Q71	L82	R04.2	R24	R16.2	B87	R25.8	N08
Q72	L82	R04.8	R29	R16.2	D23	R26.0	N29
Q73	L82	R04.9	R29	R17	D13	R26.1	N29
Q74	L82	R05	R05	R18	D29	R26.2	N29
Q75	L82	R06.0	R02	R19.0	D24	R26.8	A29
Q76	L82	R06.1	R04	R19.0	D25	R26.8	L29
Q77	L82	R06.2	R03	R19.1	D29	R26.8	N29
Q78	L82	R06.3	R04	R19.2	D29	R27	N29
Q79	L82	R06.4	R98	R19.3	D29	R29.0	N08
Q80	S83	R06.5	R04	R19.4	D18	R29.0	N29
Q81	S83	R06.6	R29	R19.5	D18	R29.1	N29
Q82	S83	R06.7	R07	R19.6	D20	R29.2	N29
Q83	X83	R06.8	R04	R19.8	D29	R29.3	L29
Q83	Y84	R07.0	R21	R20.0	N06	R29.4	L13
Q84	S83	R07.1	R01	R20.1	N06	R29.8	L04
Q85	A90	R07.2	K01	R20.2	N05	R29.8	L05

ICD-10	ICPC-2	ICD-10	ICPC-2	ICD-10	ICPC-2	ICD-10	ICPC-2
R29.8	L07	R46.8	W21	R75	B90	S00.7	S19
R29.8	L09	R46.8	X22	R76	A91	S00.8	S12
R29.8	L12	R47	N19	R77	A91	S00.8	S15
R29.8	L14	R48	P24	R78	A91	S00.8	S16
R29.8	L17	R49	R23	R79	A91	S00.8	S17
R29.8	L29	R50	A03	R80	U98	S00.8	S19
R29.8	N29	R51	N01	R81	U98	S00.9	S12
R30	U01	R51	N03	R82	U98	S00.9	S15
R31	U06	R52	A01	R83	A91	S00.9	S16
R32	U04	R53	A04	R84	A91	S00.9	S17
R33	U08	R53	A05	R85	A91	S00.9	S19
R34	U05	R54	P05	R86	A91	S01.0	S18
R35	U02	R55	A06	R87	A91	S01.1	F79
R36	X29	R56	N07	R87	X86	S01.2	R88
R36	Y03	R57	K99	R89	A91	S01.2	S18
R39.0	U13	R58	A10	R90	A91	S01.3	H79
R39.1	U05	R59	B02	R91	A91	S01.4	S18
R39.2	U99	R60	K07	R92	A91	S01.5	D80
R39.8	U07	R61	A09	R93	A91	S01.7	S18
R39.8	U13	R62.0	P22	R94	A91	S01.8	S18
R39.8	U29	R62.8	T10	R95	A95	S01.9	S18
R40	A07	R62.9	T10	R95	A96	S02.0	N80
R41	P20	R63.0	T03	R96	A96	S02.1	N80
R42	N17	R63.1	T01	R98	A96	S02.2	L76
R43	N16	R63.2	T02	R99	A96	S02.3	L76
R44	P29	R63.3	T04	S00.0	S12	S02.4	L76
R45.0	P01	R63.3	T05	S00.0	S15	S02.5	D80
R45.1	P04	R63.4	T08	S00.0	S16	S02.6	L76
R45.2	P03	R63.5	T07	S00.0	S17	S02.7	L76
R45.3	P03	R63.8	T29	S00.0	S19	S02.8	L76
R45.4	P04	R64	T08	S00.1	F75	S02.9	L76
R45.5	P04	R68.0	A29	S00.2	F79	S02.9	N80
R45.6	P04	R68.1	A16	S00.2	S12	S03.0	L80
R45.7	P29	R68.2	D20	S00.2	S15	S03.1	R88
R45.8	P29	R68.3	S22	S00.3	R88	S03.2	D80
R46.0	P29	R68.8	A02	S00.3	S12	S03.3	L80
R46.1	P29	R68.8	A08	S00.3	S15	S03.4	L79
R46.2	P29	R68.8	A29	S00.4	H78	S03.5	L79
R46.3	P29	R68.8	B04	S00.4	S12	S04	N81
R46.4	P29	R68.8	B29	S00.4	S15	S05.0	F79
R46.5	P29	R69	A99	S00.5	D80	S05.1	F75
R46.6	P29	R70	B99	S00.5	S12	S05.2	F79
R46.7	P29	R71	B99	S00.5	S15	S05.3	F79
R46.8	A18	R72	B84	S00.7	S12	S05.4	F79
R46.8	H15	R73	A91	S00.7	S15	S05.5	F79
R46.8	P29	R74	A91	S00.7	S17	S05.6	F79

ICD-10	ICPC-2	ICD-10	ICPC-2	ICD-10	ICPC-2	ICD-10	ICPC-2
S05.7	F79	S10.8	S12	S20.7	S12	S31.4	X82
S05.8	F79	S10.8	S15	S20.7	S15	S31.5	X82
S05.9	F79	S10.8	S16	S20.7	S17	S31.5	Y80
S06.0	N79	S10.8	S17	S20.7	S19	S31.7	A81
S06.1	N80	S10.8	S19	S20.8	S12	S31.8	S18
S06.2	N80	S10.9	S12	S20.8	S15	S32	L76
S06.3	N80	S10.9	S15	S20.8	S17	S33.0	L80
S06.4	N80	S10.9	S16	S20.8	S19	S33.1	L80
S06.5	N80	S10.9	S17	S21	A80	S33.2	L80
S06.6	N80	S10.9	S19	S21	S18	S33.3	L80
S06.7	N80	S11	A80	S22	L76	S33.4	L81
S06.8	N80	S11	S18	S23.0	L80	S33.5	L84
S06.9	N80	S12	L76	S23.1	L80	S33.6	L79
S07.0	H79	S13.0	L80	S23.2	L80	S33.7	L84
S07.0	N80	S13.1	L80	S23.3	L79	S34	N81
S07.1	N80	S13.2	L80	S23.4	L79	S35	A80
S07.8	N80	S13.3	L80	S23.5	L79	S36.0	B76
S07.9	N80	S13.4	L79	S24	N81	S36.1	D80
S08.0	N80	S13.5	L79	S25	A80	S36.2	D80
S08.1	H79	S13.6	L79	S26	A80	S36.3	D80
S08.8	N80	S14	N81	S27	A80	S36.4	D80
S08.9	N80	S15	A80	S27	R88	S36.5	D80
S09.0	N80	S16	L81	S28	A81	S36.6	D80
S09.1	L81	S17.0	R88	S29	A81	S36.7	A81
S09.2	H79	S17.8	A81	S30.0	L81	S36.8	D80
S09.7	N80	S17.9	A81	S30.0	S16	S36.9	D80
S09.8	H79	S18	A81	S30.1	L81	S37.0	U80
S09.8	N80	S19.7	A81	S30.1	S16	S37.1	U80
S09.9	D80	S19.8	A81	S30.2	X82	S37.2	U80
S09.9	F79	S19.8	R88	S30.2	Y80	S37.3	U80
S09.9	H79	S19.9	A81	S30.7	S12	S37.4	X82
S09.9	L81	S20.0	S16	S30.7	S15	S37.5	X82
S09.9	N80	S20.1	S12	S30.7	S17	S37.6	X82
S09.9	N81	S20.1	S15	S30.7	S19	S37.7	A81
S09.9	R88	S20.1	S17	S30.8	S12	S37.8	A81
S10.0	D80	S20.1	S19	S30.8	S15	S37.9	A80
S10.0	R88	S20.2	L81	S30.8	S17	S38.0	X82
S10.0	S16	S20.2	S16	S30.8	S19	S38.0	Y80
S10.1	S12	S20.3	S12	S30.9	S12	S38.1	A80
S10.1	S15	S20.3	S15	S30.9	S15	S38.2	X82
S10.1	S17	S20.3	S17	S30.9	S17	S38.2	Y80
S10.1	S19	S20.3	S19	S30.9	S19	S38.3	A80
S10.7	S12	S20.4	S12	S31.0	S18	S39.0	A80
S10.7	S15	S20.4	S15	S31.1	S18	S39.0	A81
S10.7	S17	S20.4	S17	S31.2	Y80	S39.0	L81
S10.7	S19	S20.4	S19	S31.3	Y80	S39.6	A81

ICD-10	ICPC-2	ICD-10	ICPC-2	ICD-10	ICPC-2	ICD-10	ICPC-2
S39.7	A81	S50.8	S12	S67	L81	S82.6	L73
S39.8	A80	S50.8	S15	S68	L81	S82.7	L73
S39.8	A81	S50.8	S17	S69	L81	S82.8	L73
S39.8	L81	S50.8	S19	S70.0	L81	S82.9	L73
S39.8	X82	S50.9	S19	S70.0	S16	S83.0	L80
S39.8	Y80	S51	S18	S70.1	L81	S83.1	L80
S39.9	A80	S52	L72	S70.1	S16	S83.2	L96
S39.9	A81	S53.0	L80	S70.7	S12	S83.3	L96
S39.9	L81	S53.1	L80	S70.7	S15	S83.4	L78
S39.9	X82	S53.2	L79	S70.7	S17	S83.5	L96
S39.9	Y80	S53.3	L79	S70.7	S19	S83.6	L78
S40.0	L81	S53.4	L79	S70.8	S12	S83.7	L96
S40.0	S16	S54	N81	S70.8	S15	S84	N81
S40.7	S12	S55	A80	S70.8	S17	S85	A80
S40.7	S15	S56	L81	S70.8	S19	S86	L81
S40.7	S17	S57	L81	S70.9	S19	S87	L81
S40.7	S19	S58	L81	S71	S18	S88	L81
S40.8	S12	S59	L81	S72	L75	S89	L81
S40.8	S15	S60.0	L81	S73.0	L80	S90.0	L81
S40.8	S17	S60.0	S16	S73.1	L79	S90.0	S16
S40.8	S19	S60.1	L81	S74	N81	S90.1	L81
S40.9	S19	S60.1	S16	S75	A80	S90.1	S16
S41	S18	S60.2	L81	S76	L81	S90.2	L81
S42	L76	S60.2	S16	S77	L81	S90.2	S16
S43.0	L80	S60.7	S12	S78	L81	S90.3	L81
S43.1	L80	S60.7	S15	S79	L81	S90.3	S16
S43.2	L80	S60.7	S17	S80.0	L81	S90.7	S12
S43.3	L80	S60.7	S19	S80.0	S16	S90.7	S15
S43.4	L79	S60.8	S12	S80.1	L81	S90.7	S17
S43.5	L79	S60.8	S15	S80.1	S16	S90.7	S19
S43.6	L79	S60.8	S17	S80.7	S12	S90.8	S12
S43.7	L79	S60.8	S19	S80.7	S15	S90.8	S15
S44	N81	S60.9	S19	S80.7	S17	S90.8	S17
S45	A80	S61	S18	S80.7	S19	S90.8	S19
S46	L81	S62	L74	S80.8	S12	S90.9	S19
S47	L81	S63.0	L80	S80.8	S15	S91	S18
S48	L81	S63.1	L80	S80.8	S17	S92	L74
S49	L81	S63.2	L80	S80.8	S19	S93.0	L80
S50.0	L81	S63.3	L79	S80.9	S19	S93.1	L80
S50.0	S16	S63.4	L79	S81	S18	S93.2	L79
S50.1	L81	S63.5	L79	S82.0	L76	S93.3	L80
S50.1	S16	S63.6	L79	S82.1	L73	S93.4	L77
S50.7	S12	S63.7	L79	S82.2	L73	S93.5	L79
S50.7	S15	S64	N81	S82.3	L73	S93.6	L79
S50.7	S17	S65	A80	S82.4	L73	S94	N81
S50.7	S19	S66	L81	S82.5	L73	S95	A80

ICD-10	ICPC-2	ICD-10	ICPC-2	ICD-10	ICPC-2	ICD-10	ICPC-2
S96	L81	T11.5	L81	T19.1	U80	T48	A84
S97	L81	T11.6	L81	T19.2	X82	T49	A84
S98	L81	T11.8	L81	T19.3	X82	T50	A84
S99	L81	T11.9	L81	T19.8	U99	T51	A86
T00	A81	T12	L76	T19.9	U99	T52	A86
T01	A81	T13.0	L81	T20	S14	T53	A86
T02	A81	T13.0	S12	T21	S14	T54	A86
T03	A81	T13.0	S15	T22	S14	T55	A86
T04	A81	T13.0	S16	T23	S14	T56	A86
T05	A81	T13.0	S17	T24	S14	T57	A86
T06.0	N81	T13.0	S19	T25	S14	T58	A86
T06.1	N81	T13.1	S18	T26	F79	T59	A86
T06.2	N81	T13.2	L79	T27	R88	T60	A86
T06.3	K99	T13.2	L80	T28.0	D80	T61	A86
T06.4	L81	T13.3	N81	T28.1	D80	T62	A86
T06.5	A81	T13.4	A80	T28.2	D80	T63	A86
T06.8	A81	T13.5	L81	T28.3	U80	T64	A86
T07	A81	T13.6	L81	T28.3	X82	T65	A86
T08	L76	T13.8	L81	T28.3	Y80	T66	A88
T09.0	L81	T13.9	L81	T28.4	A80	T67	A88
T09.0	S12	T14.0	S12	T28.5	D80	T68	A88
T09.0	S15	T14.0	S15	T28.6	D80	T69	A88
T09.0	S16	T14.0	S16	T28.7	D80	T70.0	H79
T09.0	S17	T14.0	S17	T28.8	U80	T70.1	R88
T09.0	S19	T14.0	S19	T28.8	X82	T70.2	A88
T09.1	S18	T14.1	S13	T28.8	Y80	T70.3	A88
T09.2	L79	T14.1	S15	T28.9	A80	T70.4	A88
T09.2	L80	T14.1	S18	T29	A81	T70.8	A88
T09.3	N81	T14.1	S19	T30	S14	T70.9	A88
T09.4	N81	T14.2	L76	T31	S14	T71	A88
T09.5	L81	T14.3	L79	T32	S14	T73	A88
T09.6	L81	T14.3	L80	T33	A88	T74.0	Z12
T09.8	L81	T14.4	N81	T34	A88	T74.0	Z16
T09.9	L81	T14.5	A80	T35	A88	T74.0	Z20
T10	L76	T14.6	L81	T36	A84	T74.1	Z25
T11.0	L81	T14.7	A80	T37	A84	T74.2	Z25
T11.0	S12	T14.7	L81	T38	A84	T74.3	Z12
T11.0	S15	T14.8	A80	T39	A84	T74.3	Z16
T11.0	S16	T14.9	A80	T40	A84	T74.8	Z25
T11.0	S17	T14.9	B77	T41	A84	T74.9	Z25
T11.0	S19	T14.9	W75	T42	A84	T75	A88
T11.1	S18	T15	F76	T43	A84	T78.0	A92
T11.2	L79	T16	H76	T44	A84	T78.1	A92
T11.2	L80	T17	R87	T45	A84	T78.2	A92
T11.3	N81	T18	D79	T46	A84	T78.3	A92
T11.4	A80	T19.0	U80	T47	A84	T78.4	A92

ICD-10	ICPC-2	ICD-10	ICPC-2	ICD-10	ICPC-2	ICD-10	ICPC-2
T78.8	A88	Z10	A98	Z34	W78	Z56.0	Z06
T78.9	A88	Z11	A98	Z35	W84	Z56.1	Z05
T79.0	A82	Z12	A98	Z36	W78	Z56.2	Z05
T79.1	A82	Z13	A98	Z37.0	W90	Z56.3	Z05
T79.2	A82	Z20	A23	Z37.1	W91	Z56.4	Z05
T79.3	S11	Z21	B90	Z37.1	W93	Z56.5	Z05
T79.4	A82	Z22	A99	Z37.2	W92	Z56.6	Z05
T79.5	A82	Z23	A98	Z37.3	W93	Z56.7	Z05
T79.6	L99	Z24	A98	Z37.4	W93	Z57	Z05
T79.7	A82	Z25	A98	Z37.5	W92	Z58.0	Z29
T79.8	A82	Z26	A98	Z37.6	W93	Z58.1	Z29
T79.9	A82	Z27	A98	Z37.7	W93	Z58.2	Z29
T80	A87	Z28	A23	Z37.9	W90	Z58.3	Z29
T81	A87	Z29	A98	Z37.9	W91	Z58.4	Z29
T82	A89	Z30.0	W14	Z37.9	W92	Z58.5	Z29
T83	A89	Z30.0	Y14	Z37.9	W93	Z58.6	Z02
T84	A89	Z30.1	W12	Z38	W90	Z58.8	Z29
T85	A89	Z30.2	W13	Z38	W92	Z58.9	Z29
T86	A87	Z30.2	Y13	Z39	W90	Z59.0	Z03
T87	A87	Z30.3	W10	Z39	W92	Z59.1	Z03
T88.0	A87	Z30.3	W83	Z40	A98	Z59.2	Z03
T88.1	A87	Z30.4	W11	Z41	A99	Z59.3	Z03
T88.2	A87	Z30.5	W12	Z42	A99	Z59.4	Z02
T88.3	A87	Z30.8	W14	Z43	A89	Z59.5	Z01
T88.4	A87	Z30.8	Y14	Z44	A89	Z59.6	Z01
T88.5	A87	Z30.9	W14	Z45	A89	Z59.7	Z01
T88.6	A85	Z30.9	X10	Z46.0	F17	Z59.7	Z08
T88.7	A85	Z30.9	Y14	Z46.0	F18	Z59.8	Z01
T88.8	A87	Z31.0	W15	Z46.1	A89	Z59.8	Z03
T88.9	A87	Z31.0	Y10	Z46.2	A89	Z59.9	Z01
T90	A82	Z31.1	W15	Z46.3	A89	Z59.9	Z03
T91	A82	Z31.2	W15	Z46.4	A89	Z60.0	P25
T92	A82	Z31.3	W15	Z46.5	A89	Z60.1	Z04
T93	A82	Z31.4	W15	Z46.6	A89	Z60.2	Z04
T94	A82	Z31.4	Y10	Z46.7	A89	Z60.3	Z04
T95	A82	Z31.5	A98	Z46.8	A89	Z60.4	Z04
T96	A82	Z31.6	W15	Z46.9	A89	Z60.5	Z04
T97	A82	Z31.6	Y10	Z47	A99	Z60.8	Z04
T98	A82	Z31.8	W15	Z48	A99	Z60.9	Z04
Z00	A97	Z31.8	Y10	Z49	A99	Z61	Z16
Z01	A98	Z31.9	W15	Z50	A99	Z62	Z16
Z02	A97	Z31.9	Y10	Z51	A99	Z63.0	Z12
Z03	A99	Z32.0	W01	Z52	A99	Z63.0	Z13
Z04	A99	Z32.1	W78	Z53	A99	Z63.1	Z20
Z08	A99	Z32.1	W79	Z54	A99	Z63.1	Z21
Z09	A99	Z33	W78	Z55	Z07	Z63.2	Z29

ICD-10	ICPC-2	ICD-10	ICPC-2	ICD-10	ICPC-2	ICD-10	ICPC-2
Z63.3	Z29	Z71.1	N26	Z73.6	A28	Z86.3	A23
Z63.4	Z15	Z71.1	N27	Z73.6	B28	Z86.4	A23
Z63.4	Z19	Z71.1	P27	Z73.6	D28	Z86.5	A23
Z63.4	Z23	Z71.1	R26	Z73.6	F28	Z86.6	A23
Z63.5	Z15	Z71.1	R27	Z73.6	H28	Z86.7	K22
Z63.6	Z14	Z71.1	S26	Z73.6	K28	Z87	A23
Z63.6	Z18	Z71.1	S27	Z73.6	L28	Z88	A23
Z63.6	Z22	Z71.1	T26	Z73.6	N28	Z89	L99
Z63.7	Z22	Z71.1	T27	Z73.6	P28	Z90.0	A99
Z63.7	Z29	Z71.1	U26	Z73.6	R28	Z90.1	X99
Z63.8	Z16	Z71.1	U27	Z73.6	S28	Z90.2	R99
Z63.8	Z20	Z71.1	W02	Z73.6	T28	Z90.3	D99
Z63.8	Z29	Z71.1	W27	Z73.6	U28	Z90.4	D99
Z63.9	Z21	Z71.1	X23	Z73.6	W28	Z90.5	U99
Z63.9	Z24	Z71.1	X24	Z73.6	X28	Z90.6	U99
Z63.9	Z29	Z71.1	X25	Z73.6	Y28	Z90.7	X28
Z64.0	W79	Z71.1	X26	Z73.6	Z28	Z90.7	X99
Z64.1	Z29	Z71.1	X27	Z73.8	Z29	Z90.7	Y28
Z64.2	P29	Z71.1	Y24	Z73.9	Z29	Z90.7	Y99
Z64.3	P29	Z71.1	Y25	Z74	A28	Z90.8	A99
Z64.4	Z10	Z71.1	Y26	Z75	Z10	Z91.0	A23
Z65.0	Z09	Z71.1	Y27	Z75	Z11	Z91.1	A23
Z65.1	Z09	Z71.1	Z27	Z76.0	A99	Z91.2	A23
Z65.2	Z09	Z71.2	A99	Z76.1	A99	Z91.3	A23
Z65.3	Z09	Z71.3	A99	Z76.2	A99	Z91.4	A23
Z65.4	Z25	Z71.4	A99	Z76.3	A99	Z91.5	A23
Z65.5	Z25	Z71.5	A99	Z76.4	A99	Z91.5	P77
Z65.8	Z29	Z71.6	A99	Z76.5	Z29	Z91.6	A23
Z65.9	Z29	Z71.7	A99	Z76.8	A99	Z91.8	A23
Z70	A98	Z71.8	A20	Z76.9	A99	Z92	A23
Z71.0	A99	Z71.8	A99	Z80	A21	Z93	A89
Z71.1	A13	Z71.9	A99	Z81	A23	Z94	A89
Z71.1	A25	Z72.0	A23	Z82.0	A23	Z95	A89
Z71.1	A26	Z72.1	A23	Z82.1	A23	Z96	A89
Z71.1	A27	Z72.2	A23	Z82.2	A23	Z97	A89
Z71.1	B25	Z72.3	A23	Z82.3	K22	Z98.0	D99
Z71.1	B26	Z72.4	A23	Z82.4	K22	Z98.1	L99
Z71.1	B27	Z72.5	A23	Z82.5	A23	Z98.2	N99
Z71.1	D26	Z72.6	Z29	Z82.6	A23	Z98.8	A99
Z71.1	D27	Z72.8	Z29	Z82.7	A23	Z99.0	A28
Z71.1	F27	Z72.9	Z29	Z82.8	A23	Z99.1	R28
Z71.1	H27	Z73.0	P29	Z83	A23	Z99.2	U28
Z71.1	K24	Z73.1	P29	Z84	A23	Z99.3	A28
Z71.1	K25	Z73.2	A23	Z85	A21	Z99.8	A28
Z71.1	K27	Z73.3	P29	Z86.0	A23	Z99.9	A28
Z71.1	L26	Z73.4	Z28	Z86.1	A23		
Z71.1	L27	Z73.5	Z29	Z86.2	A23		

12 Alphabetical index

This index is not meant to be comprehensive, nor to be a nomenclature (see Chapter 1). It is a list only of the titles of rubrics (in upper case) and of inclusion terms in the rubrics (in lower case). These comprise the synonyms and terms most commonly used in general/family practice. Users requiring a more extensive index or nomenclature will need to develop their own or use ones already available in countries such as Australia, Canada, The Netherlands, and some Scandinavian countries. In order to maintain consistency, this should be done in cooperation with the WONCA Classification Committee.
Abbreviations are not included in this index, except the following:

complt = complaint

/ = or

sympt = symptom

NOS = not otherwise specified in this classification

abdominal adhesion	D99	ABUSE, ALCOHOL, CHRONIC	P15
abnormal blinking	F14	abuse, child, emotional	Z16
abnormal breathing	R04	abuse, child, physical	Z25
abnormal chromosome	A90	ABUSE, DRUG	P19
abnormal imaging test	A91	ABUSE, MEDICATION	P18
ABNORMAL PAP SMEAR	X86	abuse, partner, emotional	Z12
abnormal platelets	B83	abuse, physical	Z25
abnormal red cells	B99	ABUSE, TOBACCO	P17
abnormal taste	N16	accessory auricle	H80
abnormal test result	A91	achalasia	D84
ABNORMAL WHITE CELLS	B84	ache, stomach	D02
abortion, complete	W82	aches, multiple	A01
abortion, habitual	W82	acidity	D03
abortion, incomplete	W82	ACNE	S96
ABORTION, INDUCED	W83	acoustic neuroma	N75
abortion, missed	W82	acromegaly	T99
ABORTION, SPONTANEOUS	W82	addiction to drug	P19
abortion, threatened	W82	adenovims disease	A77
ABRASION	S17	adjustment disorder, acute	P02
abscess, breast, puerperal	W94	adjustment disorder, persistent	P82
abscess, ischiorectal	D95	adverse effect cold	A88
ABSCESS, NOSE	R73	ADVERSE EFFECT	
ABSCESS, PERIANAL	D95	MEDICATION	A85
abscess, perinephric	U70	adverse effect pressure	A88
abscess, skin	S10	adverse effect treatment	A87
ABUSE, ALCOHOL, ACUTE	P16	ADVERSE EFFECT, PHYSICAL	A88

AFFECTIVE PSYCHOSIS NOS	P73	analgesic nephropathy	U88
agitation	P04	anaphylactic shock	A92
agranulocytosis	B84	anaphylaxis, medication	A85
AIDS	B90	aneurysm, aortic	K99
AIDS, FEAR OF	B25	aneurysm, cerebral	K91
albuminuria	U90	aneurysm, heart	K76
ALCOHOL ABUSE, ACUTE	P16	aneurysm, other	K99
ALCOHOL ABUSE, CHRONIC	P15	angina pectoris	K74
alcohol brain syndrome	PI5	angiomatous birthmark	S81
alcohol hepatitis	D97	angioneurotic oedema	A92
alcohol psychosis	P15	ANGRY FEELING	P04
alcoholic gastritis	D87	ANKLE SYMPT/COMPLT	L16
alcoholism	P15	ankylosing spondylitis	L88
allergic dermatitis	S88	anorexia	T03
allergic gastroenteropathy	D99	ANOREXIA NERVOSA	P86
allergic oedema	A92	anosmia, disturbance of smell/taste	N16
ALLERGIC RHINITIS	R97	ANTEPARTUM BLEEDING	W03
allergy to medication	A85	anuria	U05
ALLERGY/ALLERGIC		anxiety NOS	P01
REACTION	A92	anxiety and depression	P76
alopecia	S23	ANXIETY DISORDER/STATE	P74
Alzheimer's disease	P70	anxiety neurosis	P74
amblyopia	F99	anxious feeling	P01
amenorrhoea	X05	aortic valve disease	K83
amnesia	P20	aphasia	N19
amputation, old	A82	aphonia	R23
amputation, traumatic, recent	L81	apnoea	R04
amyloidosis	T99	apnoea, sleep	P06
anaemia, aplastic	B82	apoplexy	K90
anaemia, blood loss	B80	APPENDICITIS	D88
ANAEMIA, FOLATE		APPETITE, EXCESSIVE	T02
DEFICIENCY	B81	arcus senilis	F99
anaemia, haemolytic, acquired	B82	ARM SYMPT/COMPLT	L09
ANAEMIA, HEREDITARY	B82	ARRHYTHMIA, CARDIAC	K80
ANAEMIA, IRON DEFICIENCY	B80	arterial embolism	K92
anaemia, macrocytic	B81	arterial stenosis	K92
anaemia, megaloblastic	B81	arteriosclerosis	K92
ANAEMIA, OTHER/		arteritis	K99
UNSPECIFIED	B82	arthralgia	L20
anaemia, pernicious	B81	arthritis NOS	L91
anaemia, of pregnancy	W84	arthritis, osteo: see osteoarthrosis	
anaemia, protein deficiency	B82	arthritis, psoriatic	S91
ANAEMIA, VIT B12 DEFICIENCY	B81	arthritis, pyogenic	L70
anaesthesia	N06	ARTHRITIS, RHEUMATOID	L88
anaesthetic shock	A87	arthrodesis	L99
anal spasm	D04	arthropathy, crystal	T99

bloating	D08	bunion	L98
blocked ear	H13	BURN	S14
BLOCKED LACRIMAL DUCT,		burn, chemical	S14
INFANT	F80	burning eye	F13
blocked lacrimal duct, not infant	F99	burning feet	N05
blocked nose	R07	burning sensation skin	S01
blocked sinuses	R09	burning urination	U01
BLOOD DISEASE, OTHER	B99	BURSITIS	L87
blood in/from ear	H05	bursitis of shoulder	L92
blood in stool	D16	cachexia	T08
blood in urine	U06	caesarian section	W92/W93
BLOOD PRESSURE, ELEVATED	K85	calcified tendon	L87
BLOOD SYMPT/COMPLT	B04	calculus, urinary	U95
bloodshot eye	F02	CALLOSITIES	S20
blotches, generalized	S07	campylobacter enteritis	D70
blotch, localized	S06	cancer phobia	P79
BOIL	S10	cancer: see NEOPLASM,	
BOIL, NOSE	R73	MALIGNANT	
bow leg	L82	CANDIDIASIS,	
BOWEL MOVEMENTS		FEMALE GENITAL	X72
CHANGED	D18	candidiasis, oral	D83
BOWEL TRAINING PROBLEM	P13	candidiasis, penis	Y75
Bowen's disease	S79	candidiasis, perianal	S75
bradycardia	K80	CANDIDIASIS, SKIN	S75
brain syndrome, chronic	P98	carbon monoxide toxicity	A86
breakthrough bleeding	X08	CARBUNCLE	S10
BREAST DISORDER,		carcinoma-in-situ, breast	X81
OTHER, IN PREGNANCY/		carcinoma-in-situ, cervix	X81
PUERPERIUM	W95	carcinoma-in-situ: see neoplasm,	
BREAST SYMPT/COMPLT,		unspecified/uncertain carcino-	
FEMALE	X21	matosis, unknown primary	A79
BREAST SYMPT/COMPLT,		cardiac arrest	K84
MALE	Y16	cardiac asthma	K77
breath holding	R04	cardiac bruit	K81
BREATHING PROBLEM	R04	cardiomegaly	K84
bronchiectasis	R99	cardiomyopathy	K84
BRONCHIOLITIS, ACUTE	R78	CARDIOVASCULAR	
bronchitis NOS	R78	DISEASE, OTHER	K99
BRONCHITIS, ACUTE	R78	CARDIOVASCULAR RISK	
BRONCHITIS, CHRONIC	R79	FACTOR	K22
bronchitis, wheezy	R96	CARDIOVASCULAR	
bronchopneumonia	R81	SYMPT/COMPLT	K29
brucellosis	A78	caries	D82
BRUISE	S16	carotid bruit	K81
BULIMIA	P86	CARPAL TUNNEL	
bundle branch block	K84	SYNDROME	N93

diabetes insipidus	T99	DISCHARGE, VAGINAL	X14
diabetes, affecting pregnancy	W84	discoid lupus erythematosus	S99
DIABETES, GESTATIONAL	W85	discomfort, abdominal	D01
DIABETES, INSULIN		discomfort, epigastric	D02
DEPENDENT	T89	disease NOS	A99
DIABETES, NON-INSULIN		DISEASE ABSENT	A97
DEPENDENT	T90	disease, adenovirus	A77
diabetes, type 1	T89	DISEASE, BLOOD, OTHER	B99
diabetes, type 2	T90	DISEASE, CARDIOVASCULAR,	
diabetic neuropathy	N94	OTHER	K99
diabetic retinopathy	F83	disease carrier	A99
diaphragmatic hernia	D90	disease, coeliac	D99
DIARRHOEA	D11	DISEASE, DIGESTIVE	
diarrhoea, presumed infective	D73	SYSTEM, OTHER	D99
dietary deficiency	T91	DISEASE, DIVERTICULAR	D92
DIGESTIVE SYMPT/COMPLT	D29	DISEASE, EAR, OTHER	H99
diphtheria	R83	DISEASE, ENDOCRINE,	
diplopia	F05	OTHER	T99
DISABILITY, BLOOD/		DISEASE, EYE, OTHER	F99
LYMPH/SPLEEN	B28	DISEASE, FEMALE	
DISABILITY, CIRCULATORY	K28	GENITAL, OTHER	X99
DISABILITY, DIGESTIVE	D28	DISEASE, GENERAL, OTHER	A99
DISABILITY, EAR	H28	DISEASE, HEART VALVE	K83
DISABILITY, ENDOCRINE	T28	disease, heart, atherosclerotic	K76
DISABILITY, EYE	F28	DISEASE, HEART, OTHER	K84
DISABILITY, FEMALE		DISEASE, HODGKIN'S	B72
GENITAL	X28	DISEASE, INFECTIOUS,	
DISABILITY, GENERAL	A28	OTHER	A78
DISABILITY, MALE GENITAL	Y28	DISEASE, LIVER	D97
DISABILITY, METABOLIC	T28	DISEASE, LYMPH, OTHER	B99
DISABILITY,		DISEASE, MALE GENITAL,	
MUSCULOSKELETAL	L28	OTHER	Y99
DISABILITY,		disease, male breast	Y99
NEUROLOGICAL	N28	DISEASE, MASTOID	H99
DISABILITY, NUTRITIONAL	T28	DISEASE, MOUTH/	
DISABILITY, PREGNANCY	W28	TONGUE/LIP	D83
DISABILITY,		DISEASE, MUSCULO-	
PSYCHOLOGICAL	P28	SKELETAL, OTHER	L99
DISABILITY, RESPIRATORY	R28	DISEASE, NEUROLOGICAL,	
DISABILITY, SKIN	S28	OTHER	N99
DISABILITY, URINARY	U28	DISEASE, OESOPHAGUS	D84
disc degeneration/prolapse	L86	DISEASE, PELVIC	
DISCHARGE, EAR	H04	INFLAMMATORY	X74
DISCHARGE, EYE	F03	disease, pericardium	K84
discharge, nipple	X20	DISEASE, RESPIRATORY,	
DISCHARGE, URETHRAL	Y03	OTHER	R99

empty nest syndrome	P25	EYE MOVEMENTS	
empyema	R83	ABNORMAL	F14
ENCEPHALITIS	N71	EYE SENSATIONS ABNORMAL	F13
ENCOPRESIS	P13	eye strain	F05
endarteritis	K92	EYE SYMPT/COMPLT, OTHER	F29
endocarditis, acute/subacute	K70	EYE, RED	F02
endocarditis, chronic	K83	EYELID SYMPT/COMPLT	F16
ENDOCRINE DISEASE NOS	T99	faecal impaction	D12
ENDOCRINE SYMPT/		faecal incontinence	D17
COMPLT, OTHER	T29	FAECES, CHANGE	D18
endometrial polyp	X99	failure to thrive	T10
endometriosis	X99	FAINTING	A06
endometritis	X74	Fallet's tetralogy	K73
ENTERITIS, CHRONIC	D94	falls	A29
entropion	F99	false teeth problem	D19
ENURESIS	P12	family history of	
enuresis, organic	U04	cardiovascular disease	K22
environmental problem	Z29	family history of disease NOS	A23
eosinophilia	B84	family history of malignancy	A21
epicondylitis, lateral	L93	family planning NOS	W14
epididymal cyst	Y99	family planning, IUD	W12
EPIDIDYMITIS	Y74	family planning, male	Y14
epiglottitis	R83	family planning sympt/complt	W29
EPILEPSY	N88	family planning, oral	W11
episcleritis	F99	FAMILY PLANNING, OTHER	Y14
EPISTAXIS	R06	FAMILY RELATIONSHIP	
eructation	D08	PROBLEM	Z20
erysipelas	S76	fasciitis	L87
erythema multiforme	S99	fatigue	A04
erythema nodosum	S99	fatty liver	D97
erythema, generalized	S07	FEAR OF AIDS	B25
erythema, localized	S06	fear of attempting suicide	P27
ESR raised	B99	fear of blindness	F27
essential hypertension	K86	FEAR OF BREAST	
eustachian block	H73	CANCER, FEMALE	X26
EUSTACHIAN SALPINGITIS	H73	FEAR OF CANCER NOS	A26
EUTHANASIA, REQUEST/		FEAR OF CANCER OF	
DISCUSSION	A20	BLOOD/LYMPH SYSTEM	B26
exhaustion	A04	FEAR OF CANCER OF	
extrasystoles	K80	BREAST FEMALE	X26
EYE APPEARANCE		FEAR OF CANCER OF	
ABNORMAL	F15	DIGESTIVE SYSTEM	D26
eye, circle under	S08	FEAR OF CANCER OF	
eye colour change	F15	ENDOCRINE SYSTEM	T26
EYE INFECTION/		FEAR OF CANCER OF	
INFLAMMATION, OTHER	F73	GENITAL SYSTEM, FEMALE	X25

fibroid uterus	X78	FOREIGN BODY, LARYNX	R87
fibromyalgia	L18	foreign body, mouth	D79
fibromyoma of cervix	X78	FOREIGN BODY, NOSE	R87
FIBROMYOMA UTERUS	X78	foreign body, oesophagus	D79
fibrosarcoma	L71	foreign body, rectum	D79
fibrositis	L18	FOREIGN BODY, SKIN	S15
fifth disease	A76	foreign body, urinary tract	U80
FINANCIAL PROBLEM	Z01	foreign body, vagina	X82
FINGER SYMPT/COMPLT	L12	foreskin sympt/complt	Y04
fissure of nipple	X20	FRACTURE NOS	L76
FISSURE, ANAL	D95	fracture due to osteoporosis	L95
fistula, anal	D95	fracture, carpal bone	L74
fistula, arteriovenous	K99	FRACTURE, FEMUR	L75
FISTULA, PILONIDAL	S85	FRACTURE, FIBULA	L73
fit (seizure)	N07	FRACTURE, HAND/FOOT BONE	L74
FLANK SYMPT/COMPLT	L05	fracture, malunion or non-union	L99
flash burn	F79	fracture, metatarsal bone	L74
flatfoot	L98	fracture, neck of femur	L75
FLATULENCE	D08	fracture, phalange	L74
flea infestation	S73	FRACTURE, RADIUS	L72
flexural dermatitis	S87	fracture, tarsal bone	L74
floating spots in vision	F04	FRACTURE, TIBIA	L73
fluid on lung	R29	FRACTURE, ULNA	L72
fluid retention	K07	freckles	S08
fluor vaginalis	X14	frigidity	P07
flushing	S08	frozen shoulder	L92
FLUTTER, ATRIAL	K78	fullness, epigastric	D02
focal seizure	N88	fungal respiratory infection	R83
foetus small for age	W84	fungal skin infection	S74
folliculitis	S10	furuncle	S10
food allergy	A92	furuncle, external auditory meatus	H70
FOOD AND WATER PROBLEM	Z02	gait abnormality	N29
food craving	T29	galactorrhoea, lactating	W19
food intolerance	D99	galactorrhoea, non-lactating	X21
food poisoning	D73	gallstone	D98
FOOT AND TOE SYMPT/		ganglion	L87
COMPLT	L17	gangrene	K92
foreign body swallowed	D79	gardnerella vaginitis	X84
foreign body under nail	S15	gas pain	D08
FOREIGN BODY, BRONCHUS	R87	gaseous distension	D08
foreign body, deep	L81	gastric erosion, acute	D86
FOREIGN BODY, DIGESTIVE		gastric flu	D73
SYSTEM	D79	gastric ulcer	D86
FOREIGN BODY, EAR	H76	gastritis (incl alcoholic)	D87
FOREIGN BODY, EYE	F76	GASTROENTERITIS,	
FOREIGN BODY, INHALED	R87	PRESUMED INFECTION	D73

heat rash	S92	hyperaldosteronism	T99
heat stroke	A88	hyperemesis	D10
Heberden's nodes	L91	hyperemesis of pregnancy	W05
hepatitis NOS	D97	hyperglycaemia	A91
hepatitis, chronic active	D72	hyperhidrosis	A09
HEPATITIS, VIRAL	D72	hyperinsulism	T87
HEPATOMEGALY	D23	hyperkeratosis NOS	S99
hermaphroditism	X83	hyperkeratosis, solar	S80
hermaphroditism	Y84	HYPERKINETIC DISORDER	P81
HERNIA, ABDOMINAL OTHER	D91	hyperlipidaemia	T93
hernia, femoral	D91	hypermetropia	F91
HERNIA, HIATUS	D90	hyperplasia of prostate	Y85
hernia, incisional	D91	hypersplenism	B99
HERNIA, INGUINAL	D89	HYPERTENSION,	
hernia, umbilical	D91	COMPLICATED	K87
hernia, ventral	D91	hypertension, essential	K86
HERPES GENITAL, FEMALE	X90	hypertension, labile	K85
HERPES GENITAL, MALE	Y72	hypertension of pregnancy	W81
HERPES SIMPLEX	S71	hypertension, pulmonary	K82
herpes simplex, eye, without		hypertension, transient	K85
corneal ulcer	F73	HYPERTENSION,	
HERPES ZOSTER	S70	UNCOMPLICATED	K86
herpes zoster, ophthalmic	F73	hypertensive encephalopathy	K87
herpes, anogenital, female	X90	hypertensive heart failure	K87
herpes, anogenital, male	Y72	hypertensive nephrosclerosis	K87
hiccough	R29	hypertensive renal disease	K87
HIP SYMPT/COMPLT	L13	hypertensive retinopathy	F83
Hirschprung's disease	D81	HYPERTHYROIDISM	T85
hirsutism	S24	hypertrophy, kidney	U99
HIV INFECTION	B90	HYPERTROPHY, TONSILS/	
hives	S98	ADENOIDS	R90
hoarseness	R23	HYPERVENTILATION	
HODGKIN'S DISEASE	B72	SYNDROME	R98
homesick	P02	hyphaema	F75
hordeolum	F72	hypochondriacal disorder	P75
HOUSING PROBLEM	Z03	HYPOGLYCAEMIA	T87
human papilloma virus infection	X91	hypomania	P73
hydatid disease	D96	HYPOSPADIAS	Y82
hydatidiform mole	W73	HYPOTENSION, POSTURAL	K88
hydradenitis	S92	HYPOTHYROIDISM	T86
hydramnios	W84	hysteria	P75
hydrocephalus	N85	ichthyosis	S83
HYDROCOELE	Y86	icterus	D13
hydronephrosis	U99	idiopathic hypertension	K86
hygiene poor	P29	ileus	D99
hyperactivity	P81	illegitimate pregnancy	Z04

MENSTRUATION ABSENT/		MURMUR, ARTERIAL/HEART	K81
SCANTY	X05	muscle stiffness	L19
MENSTRUATION EXCESSIVE	X06	muscle strain	L19
MENSTRUATION		MUSCLE SYMPT/COMPLT	L19
POSTPONEMENT	X10	MUSCULOSKELETAL	
MENSTRUATION,		SYMPT/COMPLT, OTHER	L29
IRREGULAR/FREQUENT	X07	myalgia	L18
mental illness NOS	P99	myasthenia gravis	N99
MENTAL RETARDATION	P85	mycoplasma	A78
mesenteric lymphadenitis	B71	myeloproliferative disease	B74
mesenteric vascular disease	D99	MYOCARDIAL INFARCTION,	
mesothelioma	R85	ACUTE	K75
METABOLIC DISEASE,		myocardial infarction, old	K76
OTHER	T99	myocardial ischaemia	K76
METABOLIC SYMPT/		myocarditis	K70
COMPLT, OTHER	T29	myoclonus	N08
metastatic malignancy NOS	A79	myoma uterus	X78
metatarsalgia	L17	myopia	F91
metrorrhagia	X08	myositis	L99
mid-life crisis	P25	MYRINGITIS, ACUTE	H71
MIGRAINE	N89	MYXOEDEMA	T86
miliaria	S92	NAEVUS	S82
miscarriage	W82	NAIL SYMPT/COMPLT	S22
mite infestation	S73	NAIL, INGROWING	S94
mitral stenosis	K71	napkin rash	S89
mitral valve disease	K83	nasal congestion	R07
mittelschmerz	X03	nasal polyp	R99
MOLE	S82	nasopharyngitis, acute	R74
MOLLUSCUM		nasopharyngitis, chronic	R83
CONTAGIOSUM	S95	NAUSEA	D09
MONILIASIS:		nausea of pregnancy	W05
see CANDIDIASIS		NECK SYMPT/COMPLT	L01
morning after pill	W10	NECK SYNDROME	L83
morning sickness, pregnancy	W05	needle stick injury	S19
motion sickness	A88	NEIGHBOURHOOD	
motor neurone disease	N99	PROBLEM	Z03
MOUTH SYMPT/COMPLT	D20	NEOPLASM,	
MOVEMENTS ABNORMAL	N08	CARDIOVASCULAR	K72
mucocoele lip, mouth	D83	NEOPLASM, EAR	H75
mucous colitis	D93	NEOPLASM, ENDOCRINE,	
mucous polyp, cervical	X85	OTHER	T73
multiple myeloma	B74	NEOPLASM, EYE/ADNEXA	F74
multiple pregnancy	W84	NEOPLASM, GENITAL	
MULTIPLE SCLEROSIS	N86	OTHER/UNCERTAIN	X81
MUMPS	D71	NEOPLASM, UNCERTAIN	
Munchhausen's syndrome	P80	NATURE, NERVOUS SYSTEM	N76

reactive airways disease	R96	RHEUMATIC HEART DISEASE	K71
reactive depression	P76	rheumatism	L18
reactive psychosis	P98	rhinitis, acute	R74
reading difficulty	F05	rhinitis, allergic	R97
rectocoele	X87	rhinitis, chronic	R83
RED EYE	F02	rhinitis, vasomotor	R97
red nose	R08	rhinophyma	S99
red throat	R21	rhinorrhea	R07
redness, skin, localized	S06	rickettsial disease	A78
redness, skin, multiple sites	S07	right bundle branch block	K84
reduced lung function	R28	right ventricular failure	K77
REDUNDANT PREPUCE	Y81	rigor	A02
reflux	D84	ringworm	S74
REFRACTIVE ERROR	F91	RISK FACTOR NOS	A23
regional enteritis	D94	RISK FACTOR,	
Reiter's disease	L99	CARDIOVASCULAR	
RELATIONSHIP PROBLEM,		DISEASE	K22
CHILD	Z16	RISK FACTOR, MALIGNANCY	A21
RELATIONSHIP PROBLEM,		road traffic accident	A80
FRIEND	Z24	rodent ulcer	S77
RELATIONSHIP PROBLEM,		rosacea	S99
PARENT/FAMILY	Z20	roseola infantum	A76
RELATIONSHIP PROBLEM,		Ross River fever	A77
PARTNER	Z12	rotator cuff syndrome	L92
renal artery bruit	K81	RUBELLA	A74
renal calculus	U95	running nose	R07
renal colic	U14	rupture of ear drum	H79
renal failure	U99	rupture tendon, spontaneous	L99
renal glycosuria	T99	salivary calculus	D83
renal transplant	U28	salmonella enteritis	D70
residual haemorrhoidal skin tag	K96	salpingitis	X74
respiratory distress	R04	sarcoidosis	B99
respiratory failure	R99	SCABIES AND OTHER	
respiratory infection, acute lower	R78	ACARIASES	S72
respiratory infection, acute upper	R74	SCALD	S14
RESPIRATORY SYMPT/		scaling skin	S21
COMPLT, OTHER	R29	SCALP SYMPT/COMPLT	S24
restless infant	A16	scar	S99
RESTLESS LEGS	N04	scarlet fever	A78
restlessness	P04	Scheuermann's disease	L94
retching	D10	SCHIZOPHRENIA	P72
RETINOPATHY	F83	sciatica	L86
retirement problem	P25	scleritis	F99
retractile testis	Y84	scleroderma	L99
retraction of nipple	X20	scoliosis	L85
RHEUMATIC FEVER	K71	scotoma	F05

SPLEEN, RUPTURED	B76	STYE	F72
SPLENOMEGALY	B87	subarachnoid haemorrhage	K90
spondylolisthesis	L84	subconjunctival haemorrhage	F75
spondylosis	L84	subdural haematoma	N80
spondylosis, cervical	L83	SUBLUXATION	L80
spotting, vaginal	X08	SUICIDE/SUICIDE ATTEMPT	P77
SPRAIN/STRAIN, ANKLE	L77	SUNBURN	S80
sprain/strain, back	L84	suppression of lactation	W19
SPRAIN/STRAIN, JOINT,		surgical emphysema	R88
OTHER	L79	suspiciousness	P29
SPRAIN/STRAIN, KNEE	L78	sweat rash	S92
sprain/strain, neck	L83	SWELLING NOS	A08
sprue	D99	swelling of joint	L20
spur, bone	L87	SWELLING, GENERALIZED	S05
SPUTUM/PHLEGM		SWELLING, LOCALIZED	S04
ABNORMAL	R25	swimmer's ear	H70
squamous cell carcinoma	S77	SWOLLEN ANKLE	K07
squint	F95	swollen eye	F15
STAMMERING	P10	swollen feet/legs	K07
status epilepticus	N88	swollen lip	D20
sterility	W15	SYMPT/COMPLT:	
STERILIZATION, FEMALE	W13	see appropriate body system	
STERILIZATION, MALE	Y13	SYNCOPE	A06
stiffness, joint	L20	syndrome: see appropriate title	
stiffness, muscle	L19	synovial cyst	L87
stillbirth	W91/W93	SYNOVITIS	L87
STING, INSECT	S12	synovitis of shoulder	L92
sting, plant	S88	SYPHILIS, FEMALE	X70
stomach dilatation, acute	D87	SYPHILIS, MALE	Y70
stomatitis	D83	systemic lupus erythematosis	L99
STRABISMUS	F95	tachycardia NOS	K04
strain: see sprain/strain		TACHYCARDIA,	
STREP THROAT	R72	PAROXYSMAL	K79
stress incontinence	U04	tachypnoea	R04
STRESS DISORDER,		tarsal cyst	F72
CHRONIC	P82	TASTE DISTURBANCE	N16
STRESS REACTION,		teeth grinding	D29
ACUTE	P02	TEETH/GUM DISEASE	D82
stretch marks	S99	TEETH/GUM SYMPT/COMPLT	D19
striae atrophicae	S99	teething	D19
stridor	R04	temper tantrum, child	P22
STROKE	K90	temporomandibular joint disorder	D82
stroke sequelae	K91	temporomandibular joint	
stupor	A07	sympt/complt	L07
STUTTERING	P10	tendinitis, shoulder	L92

urethral caruncle	U99	venous stasis	K95
urethral discharge, female	X29	ventricular fibrillation	K80
urethral discharge, male	Y03	ventricular flutter	K80
urethral stricture	U99	ventricular septal defect	K73
urethral syndrome	U72	verrucae	S03
URETHRITIS	U72	version	W92/W93
URI	R74	VERTIGINOUS	
URINARY CALCULUS	U95	SYNDROME	H82
URINARY FREQUENCY/		VERTIGO/DIZZINESS	N17
URGENCY	U02	vestibular neuronitis	H82
urinary infection NOS	U71	Vincent's angina	D83
URINARY SYMPT/COMPLT,		VIRAL DISEASE,	
OTHER	U29	OTHER/NOS	A77
URINATION PROBLEM,		VIRAL EXANTHEMS	A76
OTHER	U05	viral keratitis	F85
URINE TEST ABNORMAL	U98	vision, blurred	F05
urine, bad odour of	U07	VISUAL DISTURBANCE	F05
URINE, COMPLAINT	U07	VISUAL FLOATER/SPOT	F04
urine, dark	U07	visual loss	F05
urine, dribbling	U05	VITAMIN DEFICIENCY	T91
URINE, RETENTION	U08	vitiligo	S99
urolithiasis	U95	VOICE SYMPT/COMPLT	R23
URTICARIA	S98	VOMITING DIG	
UTEROVAGINAL		VOMITING BLOOD	D14
PROLAPSE	X87	vomiting, presumed infective	D73
VAGINAL DISCHARGE	X14	vulval pain	X01
VAGINAL SYMPT/COMPLT	X15	VULVAL SYMPT/COMPLT	X16
vaginismus NOS	X04	WART	S03
vaginismus, psychogenic	P08	wart, seborrhoeic/senile	S99
vaginitis, atrophic	X11	wasting of muscle	L19
VAGINITIS/VULVITIS	X84	water depletion	T11
vaginosis	X84	waterbrash	D03
varices, oesophageal	K99	watery eye	F03
varicose eczema	K95	weak eye	F05
varicose ulcer	S97	weak heart	K29
VARICOSE VEIN, LEG	K95	weak joint	L20
varicose veins, other than leg	K99	weak muscle	L19
vascular headache	N89	WEAKNESS, GENERAL	A04
vasculitis	K99	WEAKNESS, localized	N18
vasectomy	Y13	weal	S98
vasospasm	K92	weaning	W19
vasovagal attack	A06	WEIGHT GAIN	T07
venereal wart, female	X91	WEIGHT LOSS	T08
venereal wart, male	Y76	wen	S93
venous insufficiency	K95	WHEEZING	R03